BECOME A

BADASS
REBEL
RUNNER

THE ULTIMATE GUIDE
TO BEING A FIT MOM
WITHOUT THE DIET BULLSH!T

JANE ELIZABETH

BECOME A BADASS REBEL RUNNER
The Ultimate Guide to Being a Fit Mom without the Diet Bullshit

Difference Press, Washington, D.C., USA
© Jane Elizabeth, 2021

ISBN: 978-1-68309-282-7

Cover Design: Nakita Duncan
Interior Book Design: Kozakura
Editing: Cory Hott
Author Photo Credit: Laeti Golden of Laeti Photography

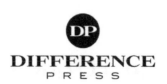

DIFFERENCE
PRESS

For my daughter, Reagan, who inspired my entire transformation journey. My reason why, my favorite person in the whole world, and my heart.

Your silly, stubborn, and compassionate spirit remind me of all that is possible, all that is good, and all that is worthwhile in this life.

I love you.

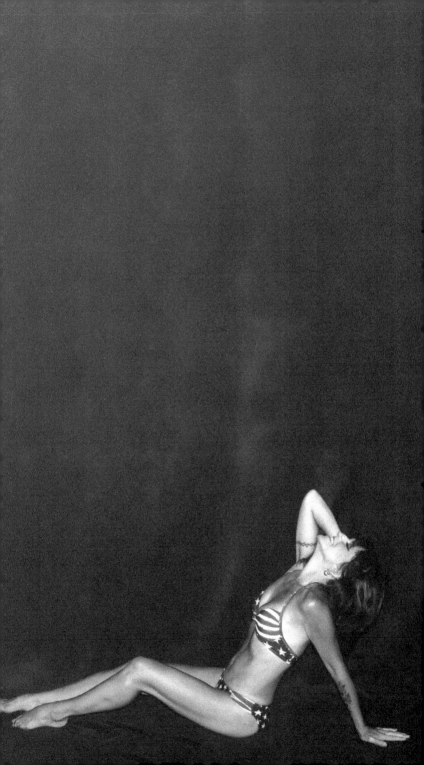

TABLE OF CONTENTS

C H A P T E R 1

You Are Not Alone..1

C H A P T E R 2

My Journey..11

C H A P T E R 3

Get Ready for the Badass Rebel Program.................21

C H A P T E R 4

"B" – Bring It On..27

C H A P T E R 5

"A" – Actually, Yes, You Can....................................39

C H A P T E R 6

"D" – Destroy the Myth..55

C H A P T E R 7

"A" – Adding Fuel to the Fire..................................63

C H A P T E R 8

"S" – Stop the Bullshit...87

C H A P T E R   9
"S" – Saying Hell Yeah to the New You 109

C H A P T E R   10
"Rebel" – Unleash Your Inner Badass Rebel 123

C H A P T E R   11
But...What If? 139

C H A P T E R   12
One More Thing Before You Go 149

Acknowledgments 155

Thank You 159

About the Author 161

About Difference Press 165

Other Books by Difference Press 169

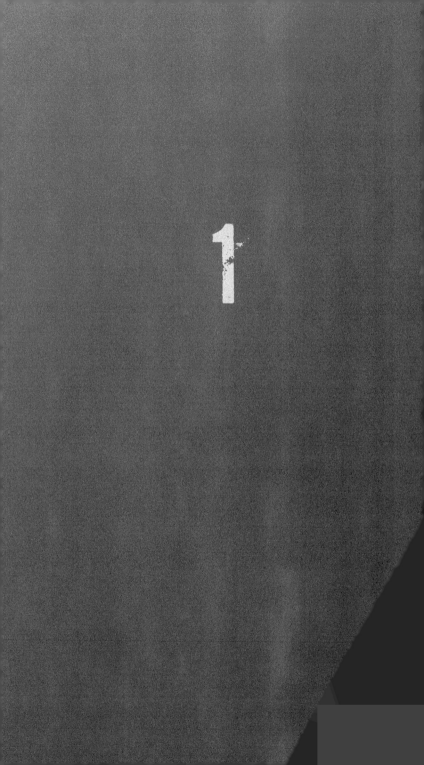

1

YOU ARE NOT ALONE

YOUR SIMPLE, HUMBLE WISH

Some people have lofty dreams of being rich and famous and flying around the world on a private jet, while sipping a glass of the most pretentious champagne available, just because they can. Other people dream of being adored by millions of people and having to pretend they hate the attention they receive, while walking down the street in public wearing the biggest possible pair of oversized shades. Some people dream of living on a private island, far away from the worries of regular, daily life, enjoying every sunset, every sunrise, and every wave gently stroking the soft, sandy beach. Okay, so that last one sounds pretty freaking amazing, but anyway, for most of us, our dreams are a bit smaller, but seem less achievable in a weird way. Why is this the case? Why is it so hard to think of our dreams coming true?

Feeling trapped in a body that you no longer recognize sucks. It does. You feel like at some point in your life you let it all go to shit and you can't – for the life of you – pinpoint where that happened. There must have been one moment, right? There just had to have been one particular trigger that made this heap of a mess that you're in right now. Now that you're here, you wish you could go back and have a re-do of that moment so you could avoid the issues you're facing. Don't we all have that wish sometimes?

However, you know that's not possible. If you had the ability to somehow go back in time with the knowledge you have now and change that one trigger, that one day, or that one moment when it went "wrong," you would change the entire course of your life as you know it. Maybe you wouldn't be overweight, or maybe you would be anyway, but all the positive things you have in your life now would also change, and we wouldn't want that to happen, so time travel isn't the answer.

Your wish is pretty simple – it's humble and sweet. You want to get in shape so you can set a good example for your children. This is amazing because you are putting the health and well-being of your children at the top of your priority list. You want them to see you happy and fit, so they know how that looks. You worry that your children will adopt the bad habits you currently have. These habits have made you so comfortable, and also super uncomfortable at the same time. You're worried that your kids will see the way you are now – unhappy with how you look – and think that it's their fault you feel that way. You know this isn't true and you want your children to know that they have nothing to do with your disdain for your own body, but you also know that they see how you feel. Kids are so insightful; they are always wiser than we give them credit for, possibly because they haven't yet been taught to turn off their natural intuition. (Side note: teach your children to embrace their intuition because it is such a powerful, impactful gift.)

You know that your children observe the way you feel about your body. You worry, and you know that you want to change things, but you have so many doubts.

Today, I know you are looking at yourself in the mirror and you are doubting yourself. You hate how you look, even if you won't admit that to people. You buy oversized shirts to hide the fat you don't want anyone to know you have. You'd love to feel good enough to wear a swimsuit so you can play outside with your kids, but there is no way you're going to wear one. There isn't a more loved, appreciated, and necessary summer swim item than a cover-up for the woman who hates her body. By the way, the cover-up is not one of those frilly, cute, see-through deals; the most loved cover-up is one that hides as much as possible. Basically, it's a loose dress that hides every square inch of fat from the boobs to the knees, so why bother wearing a swimsuit at all when you're wearing a potato sack over the top?

OH, THE WONDERS OF JUDGMENTAL PEOPLE

One of the emotions that you're experiencing is fear – not a fear of spooky, Halloween-type stuff, but an overwhelming fear of disappointing people. Everyone has an opinion these days, and your friends and family members definitely have told you what they think you should be doing. Whether their advice is in regard to your parenting style, fitness, food, education, or something else entirely, you would love for people to shut the hell up and just let you live your life the way you see fit. Social media is both great and horrible at the same time. You may say something to someone in passing, and the next thing you know, they are blasting you on social media (without using your name, of course) because they disagree with you. At this point, you just don't even want to go on social media anymore. You don't want to have those conversations with people because you know what will come next; people will either try to make you feel stupid for feeling the way you feel, or they will social media shame you. Wonderful – how freaking wonderful. Don't you just love when people purposely try to make you feel awful or like you're doing everything wrong? It's awesome (heavy sarcasm is one of my coping mechanisms, FYI).

BUT THANK THE LORD FOR LEGGINGS

Something to appreciate, however, is that leggings have made a huge comeback. I mean, you don't have to even bother with real pants or jeans because… leggings. Except, you would love to be able to wear a freaking pair of jeans and feel good in them. You'd love to be able to slip into a pair of jeans, zip them up, and button them without having to struggle or lie flat on your back, stomach sucked in, and a pair of pliers in your hands.

Yeah, I get it. Those leggings that *sort of* look like jeans make you feel good for about a day, and then you realize that an elastic waistband is not the way you want to live your life. You don't want your clothes to allow you to get bigger; you want that pair of jeans to fit – and fit well. You want to be able to go into a fitting room and *not* hide your eyes from the mirror. Whoever had the idea to put *more* mirrors in fitting rooms clearly had no weight issues because those darn things show every part of you that you would rather not see.

THE FAD DIETS, THE QUICK FIXES, AND THE BULLSHIT

You've tried all those cool and expensive diet pills, and guess what? They don't work. Those pills may have you running to the bathroom a lot, but they don't burn off your unwanted fat the way they promise. You've tried the meal replacement shakes and they taste like shit. Plus, you lost like, four pounds, but then you gained it back, plus more because you were so freaking hungry after trying that plan for a few weeks. You did the no-carb thing and you were cranky and tired, and you felt *so* restricted that you gave up. You tried the no-fat diet and you did okay for a week, but then you wanted something so simple, like a piece of chocolate, that you said screw it to the whole damn thing.

You've spent hundreds of dollars on those late-night, As Seen On TV gadgets that promise you results. Of course, they never work, and the models used to sell those gadgets didn't get in that good of shape from using them anyway. You know that already, but you held out hope that with each new fad, each new diet, and each new gadget, that this time would be different. This time would work. You'd get that rock-hard body in six weeks as the advertisements promised, and you would finally be happy. But that's not how it works. You know this already. You know there's no quick fix, and you're done with that bullshit.

BUT WAIT, THERE'S MORE

You feel stuck where you are right now, and I get that. The thing is, you aren't stuck at all – really. Where you are in your life is exactly that. It is where you are *now*. Tomorrow is a different page – maybe the beginning of a new chapter. You feel like your story has already been written, and all you can do is take a part in it as a bystander with no control, no say, and no way to change the plot, the direction, the genre, the ending, or any other part of the story. Your life feels as if you've been handed a script and you're doing a read through, but you have no say in what happens.

But that's bullshit; this is your story. You own it. You know that script you're reading? You freaking wrote it. The beauty of this is that you have the ability to change the script and to start fresh with the chapters you are writing right now. Here's a huge newsflash: you don't have to know exactly where you're going. Your story is going to go in so many amazing, beautiful, exciting directions that you can't handle reading it right now. You have to get there one page at a time, so you're ready for the good stuff as it happens.

When you get in shape, you will be able to teach your children what it means to be healthy and fit. You know your children (sometimes) listen to what you say – maybe like ten percent of the time... five percent? Ha. But they will absolutely emulate what you do, how you live your life, and how you care for yourself. There is no possible way for you to teach your children how to value themselves when you place no value on yourself.

Read that again so it sinks in. Unless you do something to change your life, you will pass this unhealthy cycle of dieting, overeating, and being unhealthy down to your children. That is a risk I know you are not willing to take. You want to change your ways, get in shape, and be the parent who sets a good example for their kids.

Here's the incredible thing – you can absolutely, 100 percent do this, and when you do, you will see opportunities you never would have dreamed of before. Your inner badass will come out and you will feel stronger than you ever felt in your entire life. Your children will love having you fully energized and ready to play with them without those tired feelings dragging you down. The things that held you back will seem so insignificant, and you will feel like you can do anything you want to do. How freaking cool is that? Your new life begins now – not in a week, not in a month, not when you "have" time, not when things are a little less busy, and not when your kids are older. No, your life begins now. Right freaking now is the time for you to start creating the life you want to live.

You are never too old to turn your dreams into reality. I know you're ready. I'm sending you a virtual hug right now and telling you that you are amazing. You are strong. You are incredible, and you've got this.

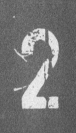

CHAPTER 2

MY JOURNEY

HOW THE HELL DID I GET SO OVERWEIGHT?

People say a picture is worth a thousand words, but one picture left me speechless. My family and I took some family pictures to celebrate the end of grad school. After months of homework, papers, and lots of sleepless nights, I was finally done. My graduation should have been a happy occasion, and in a way, I *was* happy because I had accomplished something pretty amazing. I had made it through grad school, which was something people thought I couldn't do. I was proud, and a little defiant, but when I looked at that family picture, all I could see was a woman I didn't recognize holding my daughter. How the hell had I gained so much weight? How did I fail to notice this as a problem? When did I go from having a little extra to obese?

As I sat there, I couldn't stop thinking of my daughter. She looks up to me. She copies everything I say and everything I do. She looks to me for guidance and to set an example of what she is supposed to do. What kind of role model was I for her? I was teaching her through my example that it was okay to be unhealthy. I was showing her that being active wasn't important. I was teaching her that quick meals were preferable to healthy meals, and as a result I was passing down unhealthy habits without realizing what I was doing.

In that moment, I knew it was time. I had to stop making excuses – it was time to *do* something. This was more than weight loss; it was about my daughter and her future. I had to make a change so I could show her what a healthy woman looked like. I had to break the cycle of having an unhealthy relationship with food and fitness so I could teach her how to be healthy. I wanted my daughter to value herself, so I had to learn to value myself, too. I wanted her to love her body and be confident in herself, so I had to learn how to love myself and stop being so critical of my body.

FINDING MY "WHY"

In that moment, I found my "why," the one reason that this attempt at weight loss would be different. This time I knew I needed to change, and I knew that my daughter – and her future – depended on me. I had no idea how I was going to accomplish this huge, important goal, but I knew I had to start somewhere – anywhere. I kept telling myself to take small steps each day to move a little closer to my goal of getting fit. Each food choice was an opportunity to create a healthy option, as opposed to something quick.

I'm going to tell you right now that this is **not** an overnight success story. This is a transformation story – my transformation story. I figured out how to get in shape so I could show my daughter what a healthy woman looks like, but it turned into so much more. I hit so many roadblocks along the way, and you know what? I think a lot of people would have given up, but once you find your "why," giving up is no longer an option.

At the time, I had been through a lot and didn't realize how loss, grief, and emotional pain had impacted my life. Hiding behind work, school, going out, playing out in a rock band, and just being busy became a way of life. Looking back at that time, I was so uncomfortable with myself. I was in a size "leggings," and hated it. I wanted to look cute in a freaking pair of jeans, and I wanted to feel good about myself when I looked in the mirror.

However, we're taught that loving the way you look is egotistical. How dare you love your body. I mean, really, you shouldn't show off how good you feel, right? I was in a place where I didn't want to go out. Part of me didn't want to go out because there were so few people I cared to see, and the other part felt embarrassed by how I looked. I didn't want to look at the scale because I knew where I was sitting, and from that standpoint it wasn't good. I was overweight – **really** overweight. I wasn't five, ten, or twenty pounds overweight, nope. I'm talking obese. Looking at that word right now is still a bit of a shock. How the hell did it get that bad? How did I let myself go that far into the territory of being obese?

Of course, the answer probably isn't that different from anyone else who has struggled with their weight. I ate like crap and wasn't active. Boom, it was so simple, except that it wasn't that simple. Yes, the general idea of calories in/calories out is solid for sure, but that is only a part of weight loss. I am here to tell you that the reason why I've been so successful is because I didn't focus on that part. You read that correctly. Other plans do just that – they tell you to eat less and exercise more. If only that worked, no one would be overweight.

I found the secret sauce to successful, sustainable weight loss. I did. I have a slightly inappropriate sense of humor, and I swear a little bit. I have an edge to my personality that people have told me to suppress for years, and I tried to do just that, but here's the thing: throughout this journey I've learned to embrace that part of me because she's the freaking badass who has emerged, keeps me moving forward, blocks out the negativity, and helps other people (just like you) do the same. You want her on your side. She's compassionate, strong, and a total badass rebel. I have learned to love her, and I am *so* glad I stopped holding her back.

During this process, I learned so much about myself. I found my weaknesses and chose to lean into them instead of hiding them away. When we allow our imperfections to show, there is an opportunity for learning and growing. Fuck what society says; there is so much beauty in imperfection. Some of the most amazing people in the world are also flawed, and part of what makes them so beautiful is the fact that they own their imperfections. No one is perfect, and if someone gives that impression, it concerns me because it means they are hiding something deep.

MY SUCCESS STORY (FINALLY, RIGHT?)

It's time for me to share my story with you. I started this journey at the end of 2017. Over the course of about eighteen months, I lost eighty pounds. I'm petite

– about five-foot-two – so you can imagine what an extra eighty pounds did to my body. I felt trapped, suffocated, and claustrophobic in my body. I felt like total shit all the time. People who haven't been in that position have *no* idea what it feels like to be so heavy. Going up the stairs was a struggle, and my knees were starting to ache from any sort of activity. When I started this journey, I was in the same place you are in right now. I knew the traditional diet plans wouldn't work for me because they hadn't worked before. This was something I had to figure out on my own.

Over that eighteen-month period I lost eighty pounds – about forty-five percent of my bodyweight. I went from being obese to being in the best shape of my life. When I look in the mirror, I like what I see, and you know what? It just brought tears to my eyes to type that out. It's still so raw and emotional because this journey has taught me so much about myself. I never thought I'd be okay with my looks. I thought I would have to wear those pull-up, stretch leggings that look like jeans forever because that's all that fit for so many years. I thought that I would wear oversize shirts forever to hide how big I was, but here I am, loving how I look and feel in a freaking pair of Express jeans that I couldn't have fit on one arm back then. Okay, okay

– maybe I could have squeezed my arm into them, but you get my point. I'm happy, I'm healthy, and most importantly, I am showing my daughter what a healthy woman looks like. I'm teaching her how to have a healthy relationship with food and fitness, so she never has to go through what I've been through. And if she struggles? I'll know how to be there for my daughter in a way that will resonate with her, help her, and give her the support and encouragement she needs.

Something else happened over that time period: I learned how to guarantee my success – and it has ***nothing*** to do with counting calories. I know; you're reading this thinking, ***woo hoo***. YAAAS, girl I know. This is so much more important. I learned how to set myself up for success by doing simple things each day to keep me on track, keep me grounded, and keep me moving forward. I learned how to set healthy boundaries with people who tried to block my progress, and I found my voice and learned how to use it to help other people, and to stand up for myself and my values. I learned to embrace each failure and value those experiences because that was where I learned some of the most important lessons.

I learned that failure is ***not*** the end result – it's a part of the process. The only way failure is the end result is if you don't try, or if you give up. As long as you are moving forward, you are progressing, regardless of how little or how much, how fast or how slow. It doesn't matter – progress is progress. People get so caught up in perfection that they forget to celebrate progress. In this journey, we celebrate. That's a part of my secret too, by the way. I just winked at my computer screen and gave you an air high five, so take that.

So why did I decide to write this book? You know, it was as if this book was already written. There was this force (in my head I just heard the theme from **Star Wars**), pulling me to this project. I know there are so many people out there who need to hear my story, so they know there is a way out of the misery they're in right now. Remember that degree I earned at the start of my journey? Well, that was for my corporate human resources career. As I progressed through this fitness journey, I had people reaching out to me, asking for help. My story resonated with them; they knew from my story that I struggled in the same way they were struggling. They could see themselves in my "before" pictures.

Consider these words: stuck, hopeless, helpless, heavy, overwhelmed, lost.

People who have been there need to know that there's another side to the story. There is so, so much more, and here's the best part – *you* deserve all the wonderful things on the other side of *your* story. These chapters you're writing right now are yours to fill with the future you want, and that's why I'm here. I left my corporate job, became a certified personal trainer and life coach, and created the Badass Rebel Runners program to help people navigate their way through this process, without the roadblocks I faced. I already met those roadblocks and smashed the shit out of them for you, so you're good. You've got this.

3

GET READY FOR THE BADASS REBEL PROGRAM

How excited are you to get started? You're probably a little excited, a little nervous, and probably still a bit hesitant, and you know what? That's okay. You wouldn't be true to *you* if you had zero doubts at this point. That's how you've been conditioned to think, after all. Someone has to sell you in order for you to fully "buy-in," but I'm not going to do that. Instead, I'm going to give you everything you need, right here in this book, to succeed. That's right. I am so invested in you and your success that I wrote this book for you. I'm going to teach you my process so that you can experience the same type of success that I experienced.

Why am I doing this? The more healthy and fit people are, the happier they become. I don't know about you, but I love seeing people truly happy. The higher the number of happy people there are in the world, the better. When people feel good about themselves, that positive energy is contagious. Think about that one friend you have who makes you laugh and smile, leaving you relaxed and full of joy. You know exactly who I'm talking about; you want to be in their presence because you love how you feel around them. Now imagine that positive energy on a broader scale. Believe it or not, that's what I've seen already as a direct result of people working through this process.

Annie, one of my clients, told me how this program has changed her entire perspective on life. She had been miserable and thought that she would always feel that way. She felt completely stuck where she was. She had given up all hope that she would ever feel confident in herself. When we had our first video chat, I could see so much sadness and frustration in her eyes. She had been through a lot. Her marriage fell apart, her kids were growing up, and she was doing the same job she had done (and hated) for years. She looked lost. But there was more to Annie than her circumstances.

When I first looked at Annie, I saw strength. She didn't see that in herself, but I saw it. I asked her what she wanted to do with her life and how she wanted her life to look in two years. At first, she said, "Jane, I just want to fit into normal clothes." As she progressed through the Badass Rebel Runners program, her response changed.

As her confidence grew, she sent me messages about how her life changed for the better. She learned how to love herself. She learned how to stand up for her values. She took charge of her happiness and her kids have responded in the most amazing way. They love seeing their mom happy. That job she hated? She quit. She found a career she loves. Her joy has spread throughout her family, her coworkers, and everyone around her. It's contagious. Now when we video chat, she beams. She's happy. She's confident. She has found her inner badass rebel, and that part of her isn't going anywhere.

The Badass Rebel Runners program shows you how to get in shape so you can be that amazing example you want to be for your children. I show you how to set yourself up for success so you won't fail this time. Using my program, you become unstoppable. You become a positive force working toward your goal of being fit and healthy. I also teach you how to take small steps to reach your fitness goals because it's those small steps that make all the difference.

This process is not about being perfect – it will never be about being perfect. Progress is progress. You will learn how to truly celebrate your progress and track your success as you work through this method. I teach you how to find the support you need and surround yourself with people who will provide you with genuine support and encouragement. Choosing the right people to be in your circle makes a huge difference in the sustainability of your success.

As you work your way through the Badass Rebel Runners Program you will become empowered to create real, lasting change. Being fit and healthy will become second nature to you, and you will look back at this moment right now with love and respect. The person you are right now is going to change so much over the next few months. Your future self will be so grateful for the decision you are making right now. When I was thinking about starting to get fit, I remember thinking of myself two years in the future. Future Jane could be this whole new, amazing person who put in the work, got herself fit and healthy, and felt good about herself, or she could regret not starting at all. In that moment, I decided that I needed to take that first step – I needed to do this. I had to start and then just keep moving forward because my future self was counting on me. I had to embrace everything I wanted to become in order to find the strength I needed to make my transformation happen.

Think about your future self. What does she look like? How does she feel? I can tell you right now that she is absolutely freaking amazing. She is strong. She is fit. She is healthy, and she is teaching her children what a healthy woman looks like. She is teaching her children how to have a healthy relationship with food and fitness, and she is running around with her kids because she *can*. She looks in the mirror and can't believe how great she feels about herself. Your future self is also thanking you for making the decision to start this process right now. The time is going to pass anyway, what you do with this time is up to you. Let's make the most of it, so you can unleash your inner badass and become who you are meant to be.

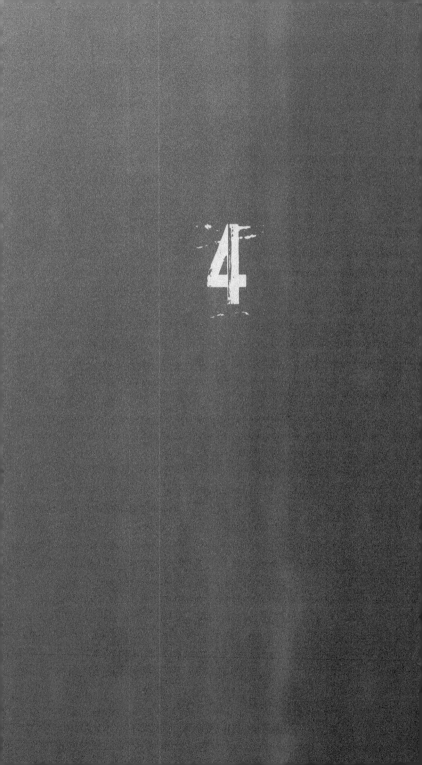

CHAPTER 4

"B" – BRING IT ON

ROCK BOTTOM: THE MOST UNCOMFORTABLE PLACE OF COMFORT

You've had those times when you wanted so badly to change something that you would have done anything to make it happen. Those moments when you really, *really,* wanted to make it happen show that the desire to change is powerful. It is. That desire, though, can quickly fade into the background behind daily life, other people's priorities, and societal pressure. Desire turns into a fleeting thought, almost disappearing from consciousness. With that, nothing happens. No change is created, no progress is made, and there are no steps forward. You remain the same person, in the same place, in the same state of being; you stay stuck where you so desperately don't want to be. I know how you feel because I've been there.

Sometimes it takes a major jolt of reality to get us to realize just how badly change is needed, and to spark the desire to move forward with decisive action. This dreaded place is also known as rock bottom. You've heard about it. If you're like me, it's a place you never thought you'd visit, let alone set up camp. When you reach rock bottom, you have nowhere to go unless you decide to climb. It looks daunting because it is. This place of extreme discomfort, this place of pain, this place of grieving, suffering, helplessness, and hopelessness is a powerful place. You see, you can stay at rock bottom because you grow accustomed to its false sense of comfort. It beckons you to just stay. It's easier, after all, to curl up and give up altogether. Rock bottom is where you must find strength you didn't know you had so you can start to climb, one step at a time. I will teach you how to take one messy, dirty, imperfect, and sometimes scary, step at a time; but with each step comes growth, beauty, and the power to continue moving forward.

My rock bottom was a place where I found comfort. I was grieving and didn't know it, staying so busy with work, school, playing in a band, and going out that I didn't allow myself to feel that pain. I didn't want to. Losing my dad at nineteen was tough. My dad was invincible, strong, and stern. He was always so sure of what he was doing and where he was going, and he was steadfast in his beliefs. My father was strict, but also kind. He was completely unbreakable, and when he was diagnosed with pancreatic cancer, I don't think my family believed it. It was surreal, but he knew. My dad fought hard, but at that time there wasn't a whole lot anyone could do for stage four pancreatic cancer. The diagnosis came with a three-month life expectancy, but my dad – true to his stubborn self – fought for over six months. I think in a way we all thought he would beat the disease. Screw the odds, we thought, after all, those don't matter – except sometimes they do.

Instead of allowing myself to embrace grief and give it room to heal, I stayed so busy that I didn't feel it that often. Ignoring that pain and that grief didn't make it go away. When my oldest sister passed away after her two-year battle with cancer, that grief popped up again, but this time, it brought anger along for the ride. I was angry, sad, and frustrated because I thought for sure my sister would beat the disease that ultimately claimed her life. My sister went through all the chemo, surgery, and radiation, and the doctors thought they had gotten everything; they thought she was in remission. In our minds, that meant she would be okay, except she wasn't. My sister was angry because she had gone through so much, only to have that cancer come back. I was angry for her too, for her children, and for her husband; once again, I didn't want to feel any of the grief that was there, and had been there, knocking at my door, begging to be allowed inside so we could hash things out.

My rock bottom was a comfortable place, without providing any comfort at all. I was comfortable in the sense that I didn't have to do any work to remain where I was. I could stay in that place forever and be comfortable – comfortably miserable. With the loss of two of my closest friends, it just added to the weight of grief I carried. People didn't recognize how low I was, and to be perfectly honest, I didn't recognize it either. I didn't talk to anyone about how I was feeling because it felt like a sign of weakness – something to be ashamed of and meant to be locked away forever, but that's not how it works.

I've never been comfortable in my body. Being a tomboy meant that I was more interested in being active than looking pretty. Plus, I was never the "pretty one," and I don't know that I cared. After losing Dad, I stopped paying attention to what I was eating. Junk food? Yep. Fast food? Oh yeah. I drank quite a bit in my twenties and gradually gained weight due to those poor choices. I wanted to believe that the dryer was plotting against me by shrinking my jeans so that I couldn't zip them up without being uncomfortable – damn dryer. Of course, that wasn't the case. My inability to deal with grief (along with some other emotional issues) had led to an incredibly unhealthy lifestyle. I was burying these issues with food, alcohol, and a ridiculously busy schedule.

FINDING YOUR "WHY"

When I was pregnant with my daughter, something changed. I noticed that the people I had been counting on for support and encouragement were doing the opposite. I was handing shovels to people so they could help me dig my way out of the emotional hole I was in, but instead, they kept throwing more dirt on top of me. These people would scoop a little dirt away, just to make me feel like they cared, but that was bullshit; people who love you don't act that way. As the time drew closer to my daughter arriving in my arms, I was trying to figure out how to keep her safe from the people who were causing me so much pain. Protecting her and making her feel loved, safe, and supported was (and is) my job as her mother. What I didn't realize at the time was that I had to change myself in order to be that person for her.

When my daughter finally arrived, the realities of motherhood hit, and I was crazy busy. Being a first-time mom with a newborn was tough, and I was finishing grad school at the time as well. I can remember wanting twenty minutes of sleep so badly. I was exhausted all of the time, as most new parents are. My daughter wanted her mom and only her mom. We bonded so fiercely that she would cry if anyone else held her. People questioned why I held her all the time and my answer was simple: that time with her was precious. As exhausted as I was, I wouldn't have traded it for anything. Your children are only little once; as they grow up, they still need you, but it changes. Forget what everyone else says about what you should and shouldn't do with your children. Hug them as much as possible and hold them as long as they'll let you. Love them more than anything because that's how it's supposed to be.

As I sat holding my little bundle of life, I thought about her future. I thought about all the wonderful, amazing things I wanted for her. I wanted her to be so brave and fearless in the pursuit of her dreams. I wanted her to be so confident in herself that she would never allow anyone to make her feel less than worthy. I wanted her to recognize the difference between love and control, and I wanted her to be able to identify good, healthy relationships from unhealthy relationships, and know that it was okay to steer clear of the latter.

In addition, I wanted my daughter to feel so powerful and empowered that she would have the drive and determination to set lofty goals. I wanted her to have such an amazing work ethic that she would do the hard work to accomplish anything she would set out to achieve. I wanted her to look in the mirror and love who looked back. I wanted her to have a healthy relationship with food and fitness so it would be second nature for her. As I thought about what I wanted for her, I realized that this was everything I lacked. All of my weaknesses and all of the shit I was dealing with were preventing me from showing my daughter how to live this amazing life by example. In that moment, thinking about her future, I knew that I needed to change.

My daughter is my "why;" she is the reason I started this whole transformation process. You already know my story. I shared how horrible I felt being an overweight, unhealthy mom. While I knew I wasn't setting a good example for my daughter, I also knew that while I could tell her how to be fit and healthy, she wouldn't get it. When children are so little, they do understand a lot more of what we say than they get credit for, but they learn the most from our behavior. That's why I knew I had to change my actions and step up to the plate in a way I had never done before. Fitness was all new territory. I had no idea how I was going to get to my goal, but I knew I had to make it work. My "why" made me completely unstoppable. I knew that in order for my daughter to have the amazing life I envisioned for her, I had to first change my life.

Your "why" might be the same as mine (except your own kids, not mine. Ha.). Think about your reason for wanting to get fit and healthy. Your children are probably at the top of that list. You would do ***anything*** for your children. Of course you would. Parents have this internal fire when it comes to their children, making them protective beyond measure. Parents can do impossible things to shield their children from danger, to protect them, and to keep them safe. Parents are freaking superheroes. When you think of your future self, are you teaching your children how to have a healthy relationship with food and fitness? Are you showing them, through your behavior, what a healthy, fit woman looks like?

If your answer is, "yes," then my friend, you have found your "why." Each time you think that maybe you don't want to move forward, I want you to think about your children. You will do anything for them.

You will move mountains to keep them safe. And guess what? This process is definitely a hell of a lot more fun than moving mountains, and we get to eat a lot of great food, so that's a plus.

ENVISIONING WHO YOU WANT TO BE

Taking that first step is the hardest part. That first step is the most unsure, the most unsteady, and the most apprehensive, and that's okay. When you feel anxious about the first step, I want you to lean into that emotion and let it happen. Be unsure and own it. Be unsteady and own that. Be apprehensive and own that, too. Why? Because, my dear, trying to mask these feelings is not going to help you. Hiding your emotions does more harm than good, and as you learn to embrace these feelings, you will become stronger and more confident in continuing to move forward. And you know what? You aren't always going to feel like you're progressing as quickly as you'd like, and that's okay. Every single day you will move closer to your goal. Some days you will do something small, and other days you will make larger strides. All of this moves you toward your goal, so every single step counts. Don't forget that.

This makes me think of one of my good friends, who also happens to be my client. She was so upset that she couldn't complete the running part of her workout due to an injury. I asked her to tell me what she could do. What part of her fitness routine could she accomplish, even with an injury? I modified some moves for her and encouraged her to keep moving forward. The person she wanted to be would keep going. Badass Rebel Runners, I reminded her, never stop, never quit, and keep moving forward even when it's tough. At first she was a little frustrated with me for not giving her an "out." I asked her if she wanted her kids to see her quit. She shook her head "no." A week later, though, she was more determined than ever to keep going. She did the work, modified for her situation, and progressed anyway. She leaned into her fear and apprehension, trusted me as her coach, and never stopped her fitness journey. That situation taught her how strong she was and that she had the ability to fight her way through anything. I am so proud of her as her coach and as her friend. This was when she found her inner badass rebel and now she embraces her power to progress through any situation.

Now it's time for you to think about how you want your children to feel about themselves. My guess is that you don't want them feeling as crappy about themselves as you have felt about yourself. Think about how you want them to feel in their relationships as they get older. I'm sure you will say that you want them to be strong, compassionate, kind, and never afraid to stand up for themselves. You want your children to be confident and brave, healthy and fit. You want them to value themselves and to always know their worth. In order for them to do all of that, you have to show your children that it's possible. You have to value yourself, so your children learn how to value themselves. Remember, it is your behavior your children will emulate, so you need to show them how to be exactly who you want them to be.

Maybe you are at your rock bottom right now. You feel like shit and you know you need to make a change. I've given you what you need to find your "why." You probably know exactly why you are going to fully commit this time, or you wouldn't be reading this book right now. You're starting to envision who you want to be in the future, and you are starting to believe that you can make this happen. Now you're ready to move forward, and I'm here to help you freaking *do this*.

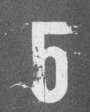

CHAPTER 5

"A" – ACTUALLY, YES, YOU CAN

LET'S GET (MORE THAN) PHYSICAL

We're taught to believe that physical fitness is just about the body. Even further, we are taught to believe that if we can get ourselves in shape physically, that's it – that's the key to unlocking happiness. Getting in shape has become all about what you look like, what you do, what you weigh, your BMI rating, your measurements, and what size dress you wear. You may care about all of those things, and that's cool, but this list is such a small part of your fitness journey. If losing weight was just about your physical body, no one would struggle because the human body is capable of being fit. In fact, the body prefers to be fit and flourishes in this state more than in any other state of being. The truth is, the physical aspect of getting fit is only one part of the journey. You're probably in disbelief, thinking, whaaat? Yeah, I know.

You are not just a physical body. You are *so* much more. For that reason, weight loss plans that focus only on your weight, dress size, and scale don't typically work. I know because I've been there, and you've been there, too. Counting calories is restrictive and outdated. That mentality of "eat less, exercise more" doesn't help you succeed. If it did, obesity wouldn't be an epidemic. The good news is that I'm here to share my secrets with you so you can achieve sustainable success. *Yay*. Woo freaking hoo. You're getting excited, aren't you? Me too.

When I think of health, I think of the whole person. While the physical body is important, we need to look deeper. For us to be truly healthy, we need to incorporate our whole being: mind, body, and spirit. If your mind isn't in the game, you aren't going to succeed. If your spirit isn't getting the nourishment it needs, all the kale smoothies in the world won't make you healthy. No, I'm not a religious fanatic and no, I'm not here to preach about what you should or shouldn't believe. So, take a breath. We're good.

In order to achieve sustainable results, we need to center ourselves. Over the course of my personal fitness/ health journey, this has been such a huge part of my success. You're probably wondering how you can take care of your mind and your spirit, right? I mean, we've been taught so much about our physical well-being, but there isn't a whole lot of focus on the mental and spiritual part. Sure, different religions have their sets of beliefs, but that rarely teaches you how to focus on your spiritual health. You can challenge your mind by learning, but that doesn't teach you about mental health. There are a few things you can do each day that will help you center yourself and help you along your journey.

START WITH GRATITUDE

Gratitude is a powerful thing. In this world of always wanting the next best thing, people often forget to be grateful for what they have. Listen – it's awesome to want more for yourself and for your children. That is amazing, and of course you want more. You want to show your children that they can accomplish anything, as long as they are willing to work for it. Along with that, though, it is so important to be grateful for what you have. Someone close to me was in this state of being perpetually unsatisfied with her life; she complained about her husband, about being a stay-at-home mom, and about the fact that she wasn't using her college degree. She also wanted to live in the city instead of in the suburbs. Everything in her life was not exactly as she wanted, and you know what? That way of thinking left her miserable. Each time I saw her, I could feel those heavy, negative vibes coming from her before I walked in the room. She felt anger and resentment for her life since it did not turn out as she planned.

Reflecting on her life, by all accounts she had it good. My friend had wonderful children, a husband who loved and supported her, the financial freedom to stay home with her children, and the time to visit family and friends. So why was she so angry and unsatisfied? It took me years to figure that out. It wasn't until I had my daughter that I realized the pressure motherhood can place on us. It is such a joy and an incredible honor to be a mom. There is nothing better, in my opinion, than being a mother. It's a lot of work, yes, but the joy that comes from motherhood is unexplainable. One idea that a lot of parents adopt, however, is the belief that their life is over once they have children. Some parents feel as if they have achieved everything they are going to accomplish in their life and parenthood is the cherry on top – they're done, finished. To them, life as they know it is over, and they feel like their life is now all about their children and their dreams no longer matter. Let me tell you, this is total bullshit.

Your life is your story. You are writing pages and chapters all the time. You don't finish writing your story just because you're a parent. Your hopes and dreams are even more relevant when you have children because they need to see what's possible. Your children need to see you work for what you want while being grateful for what you have. They learn how to be grateful from your example, just as they learn from your example of health and fitness. About a year into my fitness/health journey, I was reflecting about my friend who was so unhappy with her life, and it sparked this fire in me. I would not be that person. I refused to be perpetually unsatisfied with my life. The example I set for my daughter was my choice; it was entirely within my control to show her that she could accomplish anything she wanted to achieve if she was willing to do the work. So, I made a list. I was feeling great because I was in better shape than I had been in years and knew it was time to make things happen. The list I made was titled, "Things I Will Accomplish Before I Turn Forty," and I gave myself two years to complete the list.

As of right now, I'm not even a year into tackling my list and I only have four items left to accomplish. I think I may need to add to the list (which is already over twenty items long). You're sitting there laughing, and that's cool. Seriously, make a list, and make it as crazy as you want. If you're looking for inspiration, some of the items on my list are: get in the best shape of my life, feel comfortable in a swimsuit, run a marathon, write a book, get back into music, learn to play the guitar, write some songs, and learn to do a headstand, to name a few.

One of the most important items on my list is to make a difference in the lives of other people. That is at the top of the list, and do you know why? I know what it feels like to feel like shit. When you know how it feels to be at rock bottom, you want to raise people up, so they never feel that way. You want to send a ladder down to the people stuck at rock bottom and help them climb their way out. You want to support people in the way you were never supported. When you can relate to that feeling of being stuck, you want to be that person who cheers other people on as they progress along their journey. With that in mind, I created the Badass Rebel Runners program. What makes this program different from others is that we focus on mind, body, and spirit. Yes, I include daily workouts, and yes, I include meal plans and recipes – but that's only a part of it.

I am going to share with you what I have my clients do to start each day, which helps them get into the right frame of mind. It's simple – when you get up in the morning, I want you to list three things for which you are grateful and three things you will accomplish that day. It is so easy. Start a gratitude journal, either as a list on your phone, or (if you're like me) with a pen and old-school paper journal. I like the latter because there is something so cathartic about putting pen to paper. I feel more connected to my gratitude and my list of what I will accomplish when I physically write them out, but you do whatever works for you.

When you start the day with gratitude, you are grounding yourself in that gratitude. You will not be perpetually unsatisfied with your life. You owe it to yourself and your children to show gratitude daily because your mind and your spirit need to be aligned in a positive manner. Listing three things you will accomplish each day gives you small, attainable goals you will achieve. Since you are grounding yourself in gratitude, these accomplishments will lead to sustainable results.

Think of yourself as a seed. Alone, a seed does nothing. It just sits there. The goal of the seed is to grow into something beautiful, right? Yes. No seed wants to just sit around not growing, not doing anything, and not living up to its potential. You have to plant the seed and nourish it, and then it will grow into a mighty oak, or a beautiful rose bush, or whatever it is you want to envision. That seed represents your daily list of goals to accomplish, and the soil represents your gratitude. What about sunshine and water? Oh yes, those are all about your attitude. Your desire to keep moving forward and your ability to adjust and adapt to change as you work toward your goals are the sun and water nourishing your seed. When you are grounded in gratitude, you will see sustainable growth, which will motivate you to continue on your journey. Pretty cool, right?

Now that you're grounded in gratitude, let's move on to what you are going to do each day. Again, you need to list three things you are going to accomplish, three things completely of your choosing. My recommendation is to pick something active, something creative, and some way for you to give back each day. Did I just give you the blueprint for your three, daily accomplishments? Yeah, I kinda did. You can use these three items for your daily gratitude journal if you want to because it will make it a little easier for you to get started.

THE CREATIVE, ACTIVE, GIVING BACK CHALLENGE

I began this giving back challenge on social media and encouraged everyone to participate. The purpose of this challenge was to help people change their perspective about health. Fitness isn't just about exercise or counting calories, and I wanted to share this fact with people. You need to take care of your whole self, and this challenge encouraged people to do so; I invite you to do the challenge as well.

First up, do something creative. Doing something creative nourishes your mind, which is something we all need. The creative mind is always thirsty. You can choose to do something creative each day, and it doesn't have to be anything big. Sit down and play the piano, dust off that guitar you bought and never learned to play, and this time, invest in lessons. Get back into drawing or painting, participate in arts and crafts with your children. As you go along, you are going to enjoy these creative outlets so much that you won't want to skip a day. In fact, you'll want to add more.

Second on the list – do something to give back. Doing something to give back each day nourishes your spirit. There is nothing that feeds your spirit more than giving back and expecting nothing in return. You might think that you can't possibly do something to make a difference, but I'm here to tell you that yes, you can. Your action doesn't have to be anything big. When you go to the grocery store, add some non-perishable items to your cart and donate them to your local food shelf. Use your old blankets to create handmade beds for animals at your local shelter. Set aside a dollar a day to donate to your favorite nonprofit group. What can a dollar a day do? The answer is a lot, and this is a huge deal because people think they can't do anything to make a difference, but this is not true. One dollar a day adds up. That's $365 per year that you will donate to a nonprofit group. I can tell you that this is a lot of money for these groups. Nonprofit organizations can do so much with this type of donation.

For example, animal rescue groups can purchase a pallet of food for animals who would otherwise go hungry. They can provide life-saving vaccinations for animals who so desperately need them, or they can transport animals from the roughest places to someplace safe. Animal rescue groups can provide spay and neuter services to animals, reducing overpopulation, which saves so many lives. The list goes on and on. You may think you can't possibly make a difference, but you can. When you give back, you feed your spirit, which opens you up to growth, learning, understanding, and joy. Looking for another way to give back? Volunteer. Look into your community, find where there's a need, and offer the gift of your time.

Third (and last), do something active. Doing something active each day is how you take care of your physical body. Once you ground yourself with gratitude and nurture your mind and spirit, you are ready to get, and stay, active.

Looking at physical activity as a way to care for my body was a huge shift in my mindset. Getting active as a way to nurture my body – not beat the crap out of it – helped me see fitness in a completely different light. I used to dread working out. It was something I had to do because, you know, I wanted to get in shape.

When I started my gratitude journal and stepped up to my creative, active, and giving back challenge, my mindset changed. My mind was finally in the place it needed to be for me to enjoy the process. Choosing your "something active" for the day can be just about anything that moves your body. It can be your Badass Rebel Runners workout, or it can be something else. I love running, so that's what I do. I started running three days a week, and one mile each day. I added strength training, and mileage as I felt comfortable, and steadily added more running days to my weekly routine.

Maybe running isn't your deal. You might enjoy walking, swimming, biking, or yoga. These are all great options. Choose something you want to do, or something you want to learn. Whatever the activity, make sure you are doing something each day. Let's say you start walking because it's something you enjoy and know you can do. Walking is an activity you can do seven days a week. It's low intensity, you already know how to do it, and you can do it anywhere – perfect.

On the other hand, you may want a more challenging activity, like running. Start with running twenty minutes, three times a week, and go for a walk the other four days. When you first start running, don't worry about your pace. Start with a quick walk, and then move into a jog. If you feel like you need to slow down, slow down. You'll get to the point where you will feel comfortable running the whole twenty minutes, which is when you can start adding time and speed to your workout.

Laeti, one of my good friends (and also my client), took me up on this challenge and is one of the shining stars in my Badass Rebel Runners program. She started taking pictures once each day as her creative outlet. During that time, she does something she loves, which feeds her creative mind. She has a true passion for photography and making this time each day to express herself creatively helped her move into making this passion her full-time career. She gives back to local nonprofit groups, which has become second nature for her. She feels amazing that she is able to make a difference by contributing to these groups who so desperately need help. Her active? Well, she is a Badass Rebel Runner. This woman has risen to every challenge I've given her, and she is crushing her goals. She walks and does her strength/high-intensity interval training (HIIT) routine, and won't go one day without her workout. She has changed her life because she is doing the work. She is grateful, she is taking care of herself, mind, body, and spirit, and she is seeing incredible results.

Starting with this one activity each day will help you more than you know. You will feel so amazing after your first week that you won't want to stop. After the second week, doing these three things becomes second nature. After your first full month of doing something creative, active, and charitable, you will be completely hooked. From my experience, that is 100 percent accurate. The first week was the hardest because it was all new, but when I began again, I had my "why."

Envisioning my future self and who I needed to become – for myself, and for my daughter as I set out on this journey- helped me more than I can explain. Let me tell you about that first week. Oh, my word, I kept thinking about how great it would be for all my unwanted fat to just be gone. Snap. Just like that.

The more time that passed, though, the more I wanted to work for it. I wanted to do the work so I could be proud of myself.

To tell you the truth, I can't ever remember being proud of myself before. At long last, this was me, someone who finally succeeded in changing her life. My days of wanting a quick fix were over. That shit wasn't for me anymore. I knew all along those quick fixes wouldn't work. Of course they weren't going to work. Once I started accepting the idea that I could succeed, I felt more powerful than ever before. This was in my control, and it was something I could do. I could make this happen.

That feeling of empowerment grew over time and that is what I want to gift to you, but that's not how it works. You wouldn't appreciate the gift because you have to do the work yourself to feel that kind of pride, that sense of empowerment, and the inner fire that comes with each success. Since I know you want all of those things, I know you're going to do the work.

This isn't just about your physical body, and now you understand why it's so important to take care of your whole self. Focusing on your physical, mental, and spiritual well-being is what makes this program different than others. It's not just calories in/calories out.

I've taught you the importance of gratitude and how it grounds you so you will achieve sustainable results. The act of being grateful will bring you so much peace along your fitness journey and will give you clarity you didn't know you needed. If you do something creative, active, and charitable each day, you will be surprised at how centered and fulfilled you become. This isn't just a workout plan. The Badass Rebel Runners Program is so much more.

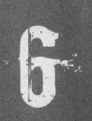

CHAPTER 6

"D" – DESTROY THE MYTH

There are certain myths you've been taught to believe. For example, you've been taught to believe that quick fixes work, that it's selfish to make time for yourself, that being busy is a good substitute for being healthy, or that where you are in life is as good as it gets, and to want more is somehow not okay. You've been taught that you need to follow along with this plan society has set up for you, living a certain lifestyle, void of anything that challenges the status quo. I am here to teach you how to destroy those myths because they are total bullshit and they are holding you back.

THERE ARE NO QUICK FIXES

You know there is no quick fix when it comes to health and wellness. If there was some type of magic pill, everyone would want to get their hands on it. Instead, you have people selling bullshit pills, plans, and procedures aimed at your desire to get there faster, with minimal to no work required. Why is it that you are willing to spend so much money on crap you know doesn't work? Are you inherently lazy and don't want to do the work? Is it that you are busy and don't have time to do the work, or is it that you are so afraid of doing the work and not seeing lasting results? I know for a fact that you're not lazy. You are so busy taking care of your kids, being there for your partner, working, and doing so much that being lazy is not the issue. Throw that one out.

IT IS NOT SELFISH TO MAKE TIME FOR YOU

Are you too busy to do the work? You might think so. Life is busy. It can be crazy busy, and I get it, but are you too busy to make time for yourself? That is a no. I know, I know. You're thinking, Jane. You have no idea. I have things going on all day long and there is no way that I can make time for myself. You may think you're too busy, but that's not the problem. You have time, but you need to find it and claim it as yours. Parents, especially mothers, have been conditioned to believe that it is selfish to make time for themselves. How dare you set time aside for just you without your kids or spouses/partners being involved? Society says this is selfish and completely unacceptable behavior, but that is total bullshit. If you aren't taking care of yourself, you cannot be that amazing example you want to be for your children. You won't be the confident partner you want to be, and you won't feel like you're ever doing enough, even though you are running yourself ragged trying to please everyone around you.

I felt that guilt big time when I started working out. Asking my husband to take care of our daughter for that short amount of time each day felt like I was asking for this huge favor. Carving time to work out felt like I was giving up on my duties as a mom by asking for help. How ridiculous is that? I forced myself to push through and think of my daughter and how I want her to feel when she has children of her own (if she so chooses). I want her to ask me for help, and I want her to make time to take care of herself. I never, ever want her to feel even the slightest amount of guilt for creating space for her health and well-being. The best way to teach her to make that time to take care of herself was to do exactly that, and I knew I needed to show her through my actions that it's okay to create that space. Not only is it okay to take that time for yourself, but it is also healthy to take care of yourself, and not one bit selfish.

It's okay to make time for yourself. You have to because no one else is going to do that for you. The space you create to take care of yourself is valuable in so many ways. Self-care time will become a time you look forward to each day. It's not that you want a break from everything else. Rather, you need to create that space for yourself so that you can fully be present in every other aspect of your life. This is your time to recharge, refocus, and unwind.

YOU ARE NOT STUCK WHERE YOU ARE RIGHT NOW

When I first started asking for time for myself, I felt guilty – super guilty. However, some amazing things happened as a result of creating this space, the obvious being that I got myself in the best shape of my life. That took time, but I made it happen. Along the way, I noticed major changes in my attitude and my emotional state as well. I didn't feel so overwhelmed anymore. That feeling of being stuck and unable to change my situation disappeared. Hopelessness was replaced with hope. Helplessness was replaced with strength. Fear was replaced with empowerment. I was making progress and I could feel it. My body was changing as I added mileage and days to my running schedule. I could run longer and farther than I could in my teens. I noticed that as I progressed throughout my fitness journey, I felt lighter, and not just physically. Feeling physically lighter was awesome, but this feeling was different. That emotional weight I carried for so long began to lift. I felt relief I didn't know I needed as I healed from wounds I didn't know I had.

I felt so stuck before, but I didn't know how to change my situation. To my surprise, I was doing it – I was changing my life. I did the work and made things happen. As the days, weeks, and months passed by, I became a completely different person. Yes, I looked different for sure. My pictures are proof of how big of a physical difference there is between the "before" and "after" pictures. What is even more amazing is that I realized my strength; the power to change my situation had been inside of me all along.

This same power lies within you. You are not stuck where you are. Your current situation is not your permanent destination. Read that again. You may feel stuck, but you're not. It feels overwhelming when you look at a number on the scale and you think of how much you want to lose, so don't. Don't think of that number as your goal. Your goal for today is to get moving.

WHAT KIND OF LIFE DO YOU WANT?

You are where you are right now because of things in your control, as well as things out of your control. Things happen in life that have such a deep, emotional impact on us that we can struggle for a lifetime without fully understanding why. How we are raised imprints habits and beliefs so deep within our being that we rarely recognize some of the damage caused by tradition. Societal pressure sets us up to believe that we are never enough, regardless of our accomplishments. All of this sucks. It's out of our control and it feels like we are doomed to fail before we even get a chance to figure out what we want out of life.

Here's the catch – you are responsible for creating the life you want regardless of all that other crap, and it's completely possible. Will it be easy? No. The most amazing, beautiful, and wonderful things in life do not come easily. That's why people settle for less than what they want – settling is easy. Settling requires a hell of a lot less effort than creating the life you want. Remember that story of my friend who was never satisfied? That's a good example of someone who settled and never made the effort to create the life she wanted. It wasn't her husband's fault; he would have encouraged her to do anything that would have made her happy. It wasn't her children's fault, either; they would have loved celebrating their mom's accomplishments, had she created the space to achieve what she wanted to do. It was always her responsibility to create the life she wanted.

Once you realize your life is your responsibility and completely within your control, you become defiant. It's like you can't believe you waited this whole time for permission to do the things you've always wanted to do. You want to get in shape, to set a good example for your children, and to be healthy and teach your children to do the same. You don't want to pass down bad habits and bullshit conditioning to your children. Destroy these myths right now. You are where all of those lies end. This is it – it is time for you to take responsibility, make yourself a priority, and create the life you want.

Now you have the tools you need to think about what you want for your future, and start to plan accordingly. Your life is yours to create and you are ready this time to create the most beautiful life you can imagine. You understand that making time for self-care is not selfish, but rather, completely necessary for your well-being. There are no quick fixes and you're done with that bullshit. I'm not going to let you slack off and I'm not accepting that you "can't" do the work. You are stronger than you know and braver than you realize. You can do this, and I am here to guide you along your way. You've got this.

CHAPTER 7

"A" – ADDING FUEL TO THE FIRE

When I look back at my childhood there are things I love and things I absolutely, positively, without a doubt do not want to repeat. There are so many experiences I've uncovered during this process that I could write an entire book just based on those memories – and it wouldn't be a great book because it would basically read like one big, bitch fest. That kind of book wouldn't solve anything, either; it would read like a private journal you write, and then burn in order to cleanse yourself from all that negativity. So, I'm not going to share all those stories with you. Good or bad, I'll limit the journal sharing to only what may help you discover some things you believe about yourself based on your experience. So, it begins.

In order for you to truly understand why you feel the way you feel about life, your priorities, your beliefs, and yourself, you must look at your past. This isn't a time to go rooting around for horror stories regarding how you grew up, nor is it the time to look at your childhood through rose-colored glasses. Rather, I want you to honestly explore all the different aspects of your life that formed you into the person you are right now. Maybe you believe that things in life are the way they are, and you have no control over anything. Maybe you believe that you are stuck doing the same thing, in the same way, and that you have no power to create the future you desire. Or maybe you believe that your current state of fitness (or non-fitness) is hereditary and you have no say in the matter. Perhaps you believe that you need to constantly explain yourself to people, or you feel like what you want for your life is out of reach. Maybe you feel like no matter what you do and no matter what you achieve, it's never enough. Maybe you don't feel like enough, period. Does any of this sound familiar to you? Yeah, I thought so.

WHEN YOU'RE TAUGHT TO DIM YOUR SHINE

When I was younger – maybe seven or so – there was a coloring contest at the local Pizza Hut. Now, I was raised in a strict household and pizza was a real treat. There also used to be this "Book-It" club in town, and when you read books you earned stars that you could redeem for a personal pan pizza from Pizza Hut. I loved this program because I read a lot. My family did not have a TV in the house. Well, we had one, but it was broken on purpose. Anyway, we weren't allowed to watch TV, so passing the time reading books was one way I escaped into a whole different world. I loved it. To this day I read super-fast and absorb almost everything I read because of that experience in my childhood. But I digress.

Pizza Hut's coloring contest was around the time that The Land Before Time came out. My sister and I both entered the contest, and I won. I couldn't believe it. I had never won anything, and I was completely elated. My sister was upset. She stomped around the house all teary-eyed and made a big deal about the fact that I won. In her eyes, it would have been better if someone else had won the contest.

I was so excited all the way home, holding onto my prize – a cute plush Little Foot from The Land Before Time. Once we got home, my dad came into my room and sat down with me.

"You know, Jane," he said, "your sister is upset that you have all these new toys. Between the contest and your birthday party, you have a lot of new things. I think you should give her one of your presents or your contest prize, so she feels better." Just like that, I went from this excited kid to a girl who felt bad for winning something. I felt like I was being punished for succeeding. Winning the contest turned into a negative experience instead of the positive experience it should have been. Do I hold a grudge based on this experience? No. I don't recommend dwelling on painful memories. Rather, it is important to acknowledge each experience for what it is, let it have its space, learn the lesson its meant to teach, and do the work to move forward.

The lesson I learned as a child from this experience was this: I could be successful so long as I did not outshine my older sister. That experience (along with many others) set me on a path of being fearful of my success. Think back to the times in your life when you won something, when you earned an award, or when you experienced success. How did the people around you respond? Did they try to make you feel bad for your accomplishments? Were they upset at you for winning? This can be so damaging because it teaches you that any success you have will be met with opposition. Without realizing it, you hide your awesome. You dim your shine. Why? You want people to like you and accept you. If they have a negative response to your success, you learn to fear succeeding.

LIMITING BELIEFS HAVE LASTING CONSEQUENCES

That limiting belief turned into an ugly beast over the next few decades. It wasn't just that one experience that caused all of this, of course, but it did play a role. I was afraid of succeeding because I didn't want backlash from some members of my family. I felt a constant need for their approval that I knew wouldn't come with actual success. I expected their reaction to be negative with any new idea I had or any project I wanted to start that didn't fall within the norm. I expected pushback, and anytime I expressed my desire to achieve something new or different, I thought people would play devil's advocate.

This negativity spread out into other areas of my life. I was always an A-student, but I was almost ashamed of being smart. I was afraid of doing better than people in school because I feared that people would ridicule me. Being smart wasn't "cool." What was cool? Slap bracelets, fluorescent plastic jewelry, pinning your pants at the ankle, Zubaz, and lots of Aqua Net, and I, the brainy over-achiever in oversized glasses, was not cool – not cool at all. The more successful I was with my grades, the less I fit in with everyone else.

In the workforce, I was afraid of achieving. I would start off strong, doing exactly what was expected of me and more, to the delight of management. However, a newbie who gets along with her boss is often criticized by her peers. I didn't fit in, and my success was mocked because coworkers thought I was a favorite for "kissing ass." In this environment, coworkers don't want to see someone else succeed, unless he or she succeeds more. I became resistant to achieving at my full potential because I knew people would roll their eyes and exclude me from team outings and parties.

On the family front, I started getting anxious and super stressed out before any family function. Without understanding why, I felt a detachment from them. I no longer looked forward to spending time with certain family members, and the mere thought of a family function made me feel so exhausted. My energy was drained before I even set foot in the door, but a sense of obligation and guilt kept me going back anyway, for all of it – every party, every holiday, every "Oh, you should come here for this," or, "You need to show up to that." I went every damn time. Why didn't I just say no?

You've been there and done that. You know what it's like to want acceptance. You sought approval where you should have been given love freely. You know how it feels to receive backlash when you dare to break away from the norm – from what is accepted within your social circle. It may start small, but this feeling of closing yourself off from people and hiding your success grows and spreads into work, school, and other relationships. You have the power to break this cycle. You have the ability to shine anyway, regardless of anyone's reactions. My love, you can only control how you behave. The behavior of others is no longer your concern. Stop dimming your shine.

SELF-SABOTAGE IS THE OPPOSITE OF SELF-LOVE

Somehow my limiting beliefs morphed into bad habits. Frequently playing out in a rock band meant that I had easy access to bar food and alcohol. I ate what was quick and easy. I worked full-time too, which I used as an excuse to not take care of myself. I was "too busy" to work out, and "too busy" to make good food choices. In all honesty, I was exhausted and just didn't give a shit. I ate fast food, junk food, and whatever made me feel good in the moment. I drank almost daily and thought nothing of it. I didn't realize how much of a downward spiral I was in until years later. Now it is so clear that on a subconscious level I was sabotaging myself. I made excuses to treat myself like crap while hiding behind being social, outgoing, and (seemingly) happy. I didn't value myself enough to make my health and well-being a priority. At the same time, people accepted me, or at least they accepted that version of me. I was invited out to parties and beer crawls, dabblers, and trips. Being accepted felt pretty good, but I didn't feel good about myself.

So how does this relate to you? Perhaps you are fearful of success because you don't want to be left out. When you show signs that you are capable of achieving greatness, people are rarely supportive, so you shy away from it. Instead, you go along with what's expected of you. You follow along with what other people want you to do, thinking that this will result in gaining their approval. Maybe you've been hiding your light and dulling your shine for fear of what will happen if you dare to show how amazing you are.

TRADITION, FOOD, AND FITNESS

Believe it or not, going with the status quo affects your relationship with food and fitness as well. Your unhealthy relationship with food and fitness is connected to a few things; for one, your fitness consists of what you've been taught to believe. Have you ever heard your parents say, "You can't be done with your dinner until your plate is clean." What did that teach you? How did you feel? It taught you to eat everything on your plate, whether you were hungry or not. Is this healthy? No, of course not. This thought that has been passed down from one generation to another can lead to overeating, depending on your portion size of course.

We have been taught to believe that we need to participate in traditions in order to honor our family. While some traditions are beautiful, others are meant to be broken. Something I was taught to believe was that I needed meat, dairy, and eggs to be healthy. This was where I got my protein. If I didn't drink my milk, I would have weak bones. If I wanted to be strong and build muscle, I needed eggs, and lots of them. None of this is based on any type of scientific fact at all – literally none of it. The idea of eliminating animal products from my diet seemed so far away from how I was raised because it was. Choosing this new lifestyle went directly against what I had been taught about food for my entire life. Eating plant-based was rebellious, which made me a little nervous. As people challenged this new lifestyle, I became almost defiant and more steadfast in my beliefs. I educated myself on the health benefits of eating this way, as well as the impact on animals and the environment. I wanted to be ready for any argument people would throw my way. This time I wouldn't let anyone push me around or make me feel stupid. Not this time.

When I first started looking into cutting meat out of my diet, I wanted to do it for the animals. I love animals, and eating them never resonated well with me. When I look at animals I see beautiful, sentient beings with personalities and souls who behave so much better than most people. They love deeper. They expect nothing in return. Harming them always bothered me, so I was relieved to see that there were other options. After looking into alternatives, it became so clear that the most compassionate, healthiest choice was to cut out meat completely. I can get all the protein I need from plants, so why harm animals when it's not necessary? We're taught to believe we need to kill animals and eat them in order to survive, but this is simply not true. Meat contains cholesterol, which we know causes clogged arteries and heart attacks. Meat contains carcinogens, which we know causes cancer, and yet, we are conditioned to believe that we need it in order to survive. Believing something doesn't make it true, and the facts don't change based on our beliefs.

At that time, I still loved dairy. Oh, how I loved cheese. I put it on everything, and I couldn't imagine coffee sans half and half. Coffee is an absolute must in my world, and using half and half was a habit I didn't care to break, but you see, I nursed my daughter when she was a baby. There is a special maternal connection to your child when he or she completely counts on you for nourishment that I can't quite explain. While nursing, you watch what you eat so your baby isn't negatively impacted by what comes through your milk supply. In my case, I couldn't leave the house for more than a couple of hours because my daughter refused to drink from a bottle. As a mother, I felt a connection to other mothers – both human and animal.

I took a hard look into the dairy industry and it horrified me. These baby animals are taken from their mothers and the milk meant for those babies is given to humans, which is then making us sick.

While I was researching dairy, that industry, and the alternatives, one video popped up that solidified things for me. It wasn't a brutal slaughterhouse video. I can't watch those. This particular video showed a mother cow chasing after her baby, who had been taken away from her shortly after birth. That thirty-second clip broke me. I was nursing my daughter and my heart broke for that mom. How could I say that I was pro-mother and pro-women's rights while drinking milk meant for that baby who had been stolen from their mom? That maternal connection changed my view on dairy, and I could no longer tolerate it. Little did

I know that choosing compassion for animals would lead to such a huge transformation in my life.

One major shift in my life was looking at food and nutrition in a completely different way. It wasn't good enough anymore to follow along with what I had been conditioned to believe. This wasn't an easy transition, and I had to take my ego out of the equation completely when researching proper nutrition. Of course, there was (and still is) the pushback from so many people who still believe that the old way of eating is the only correct way of eating. I've been called names, ridiculed, and made fun of for cutting animal products out of my diet, as if somehow that choice is a threat to other people. However, the benefits of eating plant-based outweigh all that negativity so much. And you know what? Making this choice has been so empowering. I'm creating new traditions with my little family. We do things our own way, and it's a powerful feeling.

The physical differences I noticed were immediate. I'm a lifelong asthmatic and I've struggled so much due to this illness. When I played sports in grade school and high school, there were so many times I needed to stop because I couldn't breathe. If I went for a run I would have to take my inhaler with me because it is absolutely terrifying to be out on your own and not be able to catch your breath. It's so scary. People who haven't experienced asthma don't understand how limiting it is to have to stop doing something you want to do because of a physical limitation, completely out of your control. You feel trapped and limited, and you can't do what other people do. You have to hold back all the time, and you fear even the thought of pushing yourself physically. It's scary, it's frustrating, and you want to fix it – but you can't. In my case though, cutting out animal products eliminated my asthma flare-ups.

Yeah, you read that correctly. Holy shit, right? I went from someone who couldn't run a mile without using my inhaler to a badass long-distance runner. Time is my only limit at this point. I run between seven and twenty-plus miles a day, with no inhaler and no issues. Being vegan and eating plant-based has been liberating beyond belief. I never, ever thought this was possible, but once I stepped away from tradition and the way I had been taught to eat, the impossible became possible.

I never liked eggs, so that was an easy one for me to give up. From a cruelty standpoint, research what happens to male chicks right after they're born, and you'll stop eating eggs immediately. I'm not even kidding you; it's horrifying. Plus, there are so many egg alternatives out there that taste better, have less fat, and no cholesterol. The choice is pretty simple when it comes to your health and the well-being of animals, and when you look at your food as a way to fuel your body and do what's right for your health, your perspective changes. There is a shift from eating just to eat when compared to eating with a purpose.

One of my clients shared her experience with me and it is such a powerful testament to the benefits of breaking tradition. After seeing the positive changes in my life that came from changing my eating habits, she decided to eliminate meat from her diet. She had been raised eating fried food, lots of meat, loads of dairy, oil, butter, and eggs. She had already broken tradition by avoiding a lot of fried foods, but she was intrigued by the idea of eating more plant-based foods.

Her family didn't get it. They couldn't understand why she would want to change how she looked at food. They even gave her a hard time because they saw their lifestyle as their unbreakable, unquestionable, unchanging, don't-even-think-about-challenging-it tradition. But she did it anyway.

She cut out meat, replacing it with meat alternatives and vegetables. Within a short amount of time, she felt energized instead of sluggish. As she added in the Badass Rebel Runners exercises, she became even more alive. I could visibly see the difference. She eventually went full-on plant-based and has seen incredible changes since, and I am so proud of her.

Her family will never understand why she went against the grain. The majority of them suffer from the health issues that come along with that type of diet; diabetes, obesity, and heart disease. My client's numbers are fantastic. She has lost weight, become fit, and is more confident than ever. She is a shining example of how breaking tradition can be powerfully liberating.

THE DIET DISASTER

Another super unhealthy belief I was taught is that losing weight means cutting calories to the point of being unhealthy, going on fad diets, and looking for the next greatest quick fix. That's all bullshit – I'm going to tell you that right now. In my house, we had every freaking fad diet in the book pass through our doors. All the weight loss programs (they only work if you stick with them), the diet pills, the shakes, the gadgets, the no-carb, no-fat, high-protein diet – you name it, I saw it at home. The only thing these methods taught me was that there was a desire to lose weight with no desire to work for it. If weight loss didn't come easy, it was the diet's fault and never the person's fault. Needless to say, the majority of the things I listed above are extremely unhealthy anyway, so there's another drawback.

I am going to say this again just in case you missed it earlier: all of those fad diets are bullshit. There are no gadgets that magically melt your fat away. You know those diet pills? You may as well just take a drug store diuretic because that's what you're paying top dollar to put in your body. What about the shakes that you drink for breakfast and lunch? They taste like crap and never leave you feeling satisfied. Although some of these products do have some nutritional value, you have to know what you're purchasing. Even when you do, you're not going to experience long-term, sustainable results with any of these things. Weight loss programs can work – if you stick with them. That's the key to any sustainable plan. It's you. You haven't been able to lose weight and keep it off because you haven't found what resonates with you yet, and that's not your fault. So, breathe. I've got you.

FOOD ISN'T THE ENEMY

Since I had such a fucked-up idea of food and its purpose, I felt like I was starting from zero with my health, fitness, and wellness journey. When I had my daughter,

I wanted to set a better example for her than what I saw growing up. I didn't want her to see food as the enemy. I wanted her to look at food as a means to stay healthy, satisfied, energetic, and fit. I did a lot of research looking at scientific, peer-reviewed, scholarly material so I would have a real, factual understanding of health, nutrition, and wellness. I tried a lot of vegan products as replacements for their animal-based counterparts, and then it got fun. Seriously – there is no sarcasm there at all. I have never had so much fun creating recipes in my life because I had to look at food in a different way, which meant that I was starting from scratch (no pun intended).

I made pizza, lasagna, spring rolls, enchiladas, hotdish (I'm showing my Midwestern, I know), and so many other dishes. I was truly exploring food for the first time. If I screwed up a recipe? Well, I'd turn it into something else. I still do that, by the way. At any rate, I learned how to create delicious meals filled with flavor with a completely new outlook. People who have eaten at my house know that if a recipe doesn't taste good, I'm not serving it – period. One time, I was making fried rice and the rice cooker was broken (I didn't know this at the time). I had my rice in the rice cooker and got my veggies all cooked up and ready to go. When

I opened the rice cooker, I thought the rice looked a little off, but I was so set on making fried rice that I started scooping it into the pan anyway. (By the by, you're much better off using cold rice if you want the best fried rice ever, but I hadn't figured that out at the time of this incident.) Anyway, the rice turned into a big disgusting glob of mush – gross. So, guess what I did? I grabbed some tortillas, beans, and onions and made tacos instead. They were delicious.

You're probably thinking, Well, Jane, I don't know. Maybe that worked for you, but it won't work for me. Let me tell you something: in order to make this work I had to change my mindset. When it comes to health – whether we are talking about physical, emotional, or spiritual health – we are responsible for what we do and what we pass on to our children. It is not enough to say, "This is how we've always done things." Nope. That doesn't work. As parents, we are 100 percent responsible for breaking those unhealthy cycles. It is our responsibility to show our children how to live a healthy, fit, sustainable life through our actions.

I realized that so many things I had believed about myself, success, and health came from some unhealthy situations. Likewise, the way you have failed in your health and fitness in the past has to do with what you've been taught about yourself over the years – it has to do with what you believe about yourself. Some of your beliefs stem from how you've been treated throughout your life. If you feel like you will be ridiculed for not eating everything off your plate or passing on that piece of pie after dinner, you already know this is an unhealthy mindset. Likewise, if you feel like you will be harassed for choosing to eat a different way than you were raised, just know that this is an unhealthy, unsupportive reaction from those people (and completely unacceptable). If you feel like food will fill an emotional void, you know this is unhealthy. You already know you do not want to raise your children with the limiting beliefs you have about food. You already know that you need to change your beliefs and your behavior, so your children don't have to deal with the same issues you have. As a parent, you want more for your children. You want them to have more love, more confidence, more opportunities, and more success. Of course you do. Here's my question for you: why do you feel unworthy of having more of these things for yourself?

I am teaching you how to break that cycle, my friend. This is where it ends. You are no longer going to allow your past to hold you back from breaking through that barrier you've been so afraid to approach.

You are not going to follow traditions that no longer serve your purpose, and you are done with the idea that fitting in is somehow more valuable than your worth. Is this mindset change going to be scary? Hell, yeah, it will be. The best things in life are scary at first. Think about having your first child. Oh, my word, I was terrified of doing everything wrong, but you know what? I figured it out, just like you figured it out. When you stop giving yourself an "out" you just do it because you have to. That's how it works, and one step at a time, one goal at a time, and one healthy meal at a time, you will notice that you are able to meet these mile markers and achieve success.

SETTING YOURSELF UP FOR SUCCESS

One of the main things you can do in order to guarantee your success from a health standpoint is to give yourself healthy options. Having healthy food available on-hand creates an environment that will help you make good choices. Setting yourself up for success seems so easy because it is so easy. One way you can do this is to meal prep for the week, so you have healthy, pre-made meal options. Having healthy, nutritious snacks available is another important part of this journey. When you're hungry and you reach for something, it's going to be a good, healthy snack, and not something that's going to throw you off track. Make sure you have meals you enjoy because none of this wellness journey is meant to be a punishment. You are not restricting what you eat, but rather, you are looking at food in a different way. Allow yourself to have that piece of dark chocolate here and there without feeling guilty. Bake up those homemade, crispy potato bites because they're delicious, and we're not cutting carbs. Be the parent you want your children to emulate. You don't want them going hungry for the sake of weight loss, so you shouldn't do that either. Plus, you don't need to. You can be full of amazing food and feel great and lose the weight you want to lose. You don't have to choose between those things. Pretty cool, right?

Another thing I want you to do is set aside time to be active. This is your time for you. This is not a punishment. It is the time you need for self-care. When you create space to be active, it becomes a part of your daily routine. Your body craves it. You will notice the difference in your physical appearance, yes. What is even more impressive is the changes you will experience in your attitude, energy level, and mental clarity. When you work out, your body does this cool thing where it releases endorphins. This makes you feel good, which is why your body craves more. Instead of craving fried food and sugary drinks, you will get to the point where you look forward to your daily workout routine. You set yourself up for success by making the time to be active every single day. No excuses.

When you take a step back and explore the reasons why you are accepting less than what you deserve in life, you can destroy the shit out of those myths. You are not bound to traditions that do not serve your best interests. Food is fuel to help your body thrive while you become the healthy, fit mom you've always wanted to be. I taught you how to set yourself up for success so you can avoid all the pitfalls that used to break you. You know that no matter what, you are born to shine and fitting in is completely useless. There are no excuses this time around. You are worth so much more.

8

"S" – STOP THE BULLSHIT

CHECK YOURSELF AND YOUR CIRCLE

If your circle isn't supporting you, you need to reassess the people with whom you associate. Read that again. Who do you include in your circle? Who has a right to be there? I know what you've been taught, and you already know I'm going to tell you it's bullshit. No one has an automatic right to be in your circle. You choose who is in your circle, who is on the outskirts of your circle, and who you cut out of your life altogether. You make that decision. I will tell you right now that as you progress in your fitness and wellness journey, your circle will change. Some people who you thought would be there for you and would be so happy for your success will fall away, drift away, hell – some of them will run away. Some people you thought would be so supportive will turn against you. That's how success looks, my dear. A lot of people can't handle seeing others succeed. What we are going to do is find those people who are truly supportive, and we are going to nourish those relationships. After you succeed, and you take a look at the people who turned against you, you may want to cut them out of your life, or at the least, create boundaries and limit your interactions with them.

When you think of support, what comes to mind? Do you think of a certain someone? Does a feeling take over your emotions and make you feel all warm and fuzzy? Or are you sitting there thinking, Gosh, I wish I knew what real support feels like. I get it – all of it. We've been conditioned to believe that certain people – certain relationships – automatically come with support and encouragement. This is so often not the case. Children do not know limits until limits are taught to them. Sometimes this is a good thing; from a safety standpoint, obviously you want your child to understand limits. You want children to know and embrace healthy limits when it comes to their interactions with others because you don't want your child believing every person out there is safe. As adults, we know that there are horrible people in the world, and we have to teach our children how to set healthy limits in order to keep them safe. There are speed limits on (most) roads to keep us safe. There are weight limits for elevators, rides, and a host of other things to ensure mechanisms don't overload and crash. Limits are sometimes necessary and good. That being said, there are limiting beliefs that are unnecessary and detrimental to our growth.

Did you ever come up with a super fantastic, super fabulous idea and get super excited about it? Of course, you have. What happened with that idea? Did you talk to someone about it? What was their reaction? Perhaps you can relate to this. Let's consider what often happens when you have a new, great idea: you have this super fabulous idea and you get super-duper excited. This idea is so freaking cool and you can't wait to share it with someone. You tell someone your amazing idea and then, guess what? That person pops that balloon of excitement by making a statement of limiting belief. The list is endless, and I'm sure you can fill in what people have said to you from your own experience:

- "Well, that won't happen because…"
- "Do you actually think you can pull that off?"
- "That's a stupid idea."
- "Yeah I think I saw that someone else did that already."

And yet, even though the wind has been knocked out of your sails, you keep going back to this person when you have great ideas. Each time, you feel defeated before you even *start* turning your great ideas into reality. Why? This person is probably someone close to you. Maybe this person is a family member or close friend, and because he or she is close in relation to you, or is someone you've known a long time, you believe that you will receive support. You believe that this person wants you to succeed, will encourage you, and wants you to be happy, but he or she does the opposite. Negative people like this don't support you, they don't believe in you, and they absolutely do not want to see you succeed. If you've experienced this in your life, it's time to reassess your circle.

I allowed this to happen for the majority of my life until I recognized this unhealthy cycle of limiting beliefs. I would get a super-duper fantastic idea, get all excited about it, and even come up with a plan to make it happen. I knew that this plan would work, and I fully believed in myself, the idea, and the plan. The result was going to be awesome, but just like every time before, I would go and share this excitement with one person who would immediately shut it down with statements of limiting belief. So why did I keep going back to her? Why did I share things when she was clearly not supportive? Well, that's where conditioning comes into play. You're probably sitting there thinking, Oh my word, I know exactly how this feels. I've been there, and I don't even know what the hell I'm supposed to do.

It's okay. I've got you. I will teach you how to surround yourself with supportive, amazing people who love seeing you succeed.

SETTING HEALTHY BOUNDARIES IS OKAY AND NECESSARY

Setting boundaries has taken me most of my life to figure out, but now that I've got it, I want to share it with the world. I want to be that person who tells you that it's okay to stop sharing your amazing ideas with people who "cut you down to size." That's exactly what they are doing. When people tell you that you can't possibly do something, it has nothing to do with you. Read that again, and read it as many freaking times as you need to in order for it to sink in. Seriously, read it again. Other people have absolutely no right to make you feel like you are "less than." Here's what I mean – someone may tell you that you aren't good enough. They may say you aren't smart enough, pretty enough, educated enough, connected enough, or just plain not enough. None of these things are true. These people suck, and I wish that I could just jump in and run interference for you so that you could know what it's like to have someone have your back. However, that wouldn't help you in the long run. You have to be the one to do the work.

It's super scary to think about standing up to this person. Why? Because they have been systematically making you feel inferior for a long time, and they've been successful – until now. Now is the time for you to learn how to set healthy boundaries. It doesn't matter who someone is, how long you've known them, or what relation they are to you. What does matter is his or her behavior. As you go along in your fitness journey, these negative people will try to make you feel like you can't succeed, or they may gossip about you behind your back. You may feel isolated from a lot of people as you become a healthier, stronger version of yourself. Why? When these people are no longer able to control your emotions, they are probably going to back away from you. When they learn that they can no longer control you, they lose interest in you pretty quickly.

I can tell you from experience that when I started setting boundaries with people, I felt completely isolated. I received nasty text messages like, I can't believe you would exclude me from this decision. What the hell is wrong with you? It's interesting to see the reaction from toxic people once you stop playing their game. It isn't easy because these people are good at what they do.

Toxic people may try to make you feel safe from time to time just so they can clobber you once again with their limiting beliefs. One of the worst parts of this whole thing is that most of the time these toxic relationships are close to us – really close.

What does a toxic relationship look like? It can involve anyone – including friends or family. The sucky part is that these people are often really close to us, so recognizing that the relationship is toxic can be hard. Setting boundaries is even more difficult, but the freedom you experience once you've got it down is amazing and absolutely worth it. Okay, so how do you know if a relationship is toxic? This answer will vary from person to person, but what I like to do is ask clients how they feel around certain people. When you get a text message from this person do you immediately tense up? You know exactly what I mean. You see their name come across your phone and you don't even want to look at the message. The text could be something simple like an invite to a party, but you don't even want to look at it. There is a reason you feel that way. Listen to your instincts. Trust your intuition. Intuition is a gift, and you have this gift for a reason, so use it. Is it normal to be stressed out when you merely think of interacting with someone? No. Your body is responding to what it already knows is a bad situation.

These toxic people will try to control your time as well. They will want to get together with you and will push and push and push – until you give in and say yes. When you do see this person, you may think, oh, this isn't too bad. They are being nice to me today. Wait. What? It should never be the exception to the rule that people treat you with respect; that should be the default. When you are with toxic people, they may be nice to you sometimes. Yes, they will treat you well sometimes by design. This "kindness" softens you up, so you let your guard down. Then this person will say something to make you feel bad about yourself or your situation, or they may try to make you feel guilty for your accomplishments. Behind your back, he or she may trash talk you to other people.

Let's stop on this point for one minute. There are two prongs to gossip: the person gossiping and the person allowing the gossip to happen. Don't be either of those prongs. Gossip is a vicious tool used by weak people to manipulate, control, and isolate others; it is unkind, uncool, and unnecessary. If someone is gossiping to you about someone else, I guarantee that he or she is doing the same about you behind your back. Stop that cycle now and take out the trash. When someone starts that crap, you can say something like, "I'm not participating in this conversation." Shut it down. Once I started doing that, some people stopped talking to me, which was surprisingly liberating. They still talk about me behind my back, but that's okay. Clearly, they are impacted by what I'm doing so much that they are stalking my social media pages and talking about me. They're obviously fans of mine.

When you create boundaries, it will be a little scary because you are breaking the cycle of emotional abuse with these toxic people. People who constantly put you down, make you feel small, tell you that you aren't enough, gossip about you, turn others against you, and try to make you feel like you aren't enough are abusive from an emotional standpoint. One comment one time does not put someone in this category; it's the consistent, persistent, negative bullshit that weighs you down and crushes your spirit. It's time, my love – time to break that cycle.

CHOOSING HEALTHY RELATIONSHIPS

Let me tell you what doesn't matter in relationships:
- The length of time you've known someone
- Being related through blood or marriage
- How you met someone

What does matter? The health of the relationship. Not every "not so great" relationship is toxic. Sometimes there are people who just don't mesh with you;

your personalities don't click, and that's okay. Not connecting doesn't make these people bad and it doesn't make those relationships toxic. I mean, do you want to spend your time with someone who doesn't gel with you? Probably not often. However, these people can be important because if they are good people and want the best for you, it doesn't matter if you have a weekly coffee date, just keep in touch through social media, or see them every now and then. These people play an important role in your life.

Let me give you an example of the kind of relationship I'm talking about. I've known several people over the years who are good people, but for whatever reason our personalities just don't quite mesh. Now, I can talk to anyone. I'm outgoing and have no issues carrying on a conversation, but that doesn't mean I'm always comfortable with everyone. I have a friend who I've known for almost two decades. He's a nice person and we get along, but he isn't someone I'd want to hang out with often. We just don't click, but we are friends and we support each other anyway. You don't have to be super close and cozy with everyone in your life. It's not even possible.

IT AIN'T WRONG TO WANT IT TO BE RIGHT

Let's chat about setting boundaries. When I first started doing this it felt so weird and so awkward. Setting boundaries felt like I was doing something wrong. Don't worry about that because all of those feelings are remnants of that damn conditioning you are going to leave behind. I am showing you how to break that cycle so your children aren't restricted by the limiting beliefs you've been taught. You thought those beliefs were fine, but those beliefs held you back and never felt quite right. I am teaching you how to break that cycle, so you feel the freedom of making your own damn decisions without obligation on one shoulder and guilt on the other.

I want you to start by setting your priorities. What do you want to accomplish? You already know that you need to make time for yourself. You need to have that time to be active and take care of yourself. You need to create space for self-care. You want to spend time with your children, of course, and you may have work that needs to get done, so that goes on the list too. Make your "have-to-do" list as well as a list of things you want to do. Your priorities, surprisingly enough, will come from both of these lists. What you don't need to do is anything that does not serve your purpose. Additionally, keep the things you need to do and the things you want to do in mind when people ask you to make time for other things.

Stacy, one of my dear clients, was invited to a party and she felt obligated to go. She reached out to me because she didn't want to go and she wasn't confident in her "no." I asked her to break it down from a time standpoint. This party was a big commitment – it would take her an hour or so to get ready for that party, at least a half-hour to drive there, a couple of hours or more to spend time at the event, another half-hour to drive home, and then time to decompress. All in all, this seemingly simple party would take up at least five hours of her day. Now, if she wanted to go, she wouldn't have had an issue with this. But she didn't want to go. Even though she felt obligated to be there, she had her list of priorities set for the day. She had things she had to do and things she wanted to do. In that five-plus hour timeframe, she wanted to have the freedom to do what was important to her instead of giving into social obligation. I asked her why she felt so guilty for wanting to say no. "Jane," she said, "I don't know. I'm just so used to doing what everyone else wants me to do."

"Stacy," I replied, "I am here to tell you that it is okay to say no. It is okay to tell your friend no without overexplaining why you aren't going to their party. You have things you want to do and now is the time for you to make those things a priority over what other people want you to do." I could hear relief in her voice as she thanked me. She was waiting for permission to say no. This stops here and now. Permission is never required to make time for your priorities.

The same goes for that friend or family member who "just wants to meet for drinks." If you want to go, by all means go, but don't go out of obligation. The dilemma of family functions will come up as well. Do you want to go? Is your family kind to you? If yes, then go. Absolutely make time for your family, but if they are not kind to you and you leave each family function stressed out and anxious, it's okay to say no. This is probably one of the hardest situations because of the "but we're family" argument and the guilt trips that inherently go along with family. Just because someone is related to you doesn't give them free and unlimited access to your time. You decide how to spend your time. And don't you dare feel guilty for saying no.

GUILT TRIP BLOCKER

I've come to realize that a huge factor in how I've allowed myself to be treated over the years has to do with guilt. There is a built-in mechanism that is triggered when I think of saying "no" to certain people and certain situations. A nagging feeling of impending regret and ultimate doom pops up if I don't follow along with what I've been conditioned to believe.

The truth is, guilt should never play a role in your decision-making process. Guilt makes you second guess what you know to be true and it makes you doubt yourself, your worth, and your convictions. I do something so simple when I start to feel that nagging guilt (or when someone tries to guilt-trip me). I physically put my hand up (think "Stop! In the Name of Love") and I say, "Fuck that." You don't have to swear if you don't want to. You can say, "no," or "screw that," or "not this time," or whatever works for you. This is so freaking simple and so freaking powerful. That physical action combined with you verbally saying no to the guilt trip is beyond empowering. Try it, right now. Try it. I'm sure you feel a little awkward at first, probably. But you smiled, didn't you? Hell, yeah. Now every single time guilt gets in your way, I want you to do this exercise and you will be surprised at how great it feels.

FINDING THE SUPPORT YOU NEED

What does real support look like? Think back to a time when you felt like you could do anything, when you thought, This is going to work this time and I know this person has my back. For you, this exploration won't be exactly like mine. Either way, there is no wrong answer. Seriously, I'm not going to go in and correct your memories or tell you you're wrong. My guess is that you've heard that enough in your life and it's time you allow yourself to simply embrace your past – the good parts and the shitty parts. Think back to a moment when you first thought you were not good enough. Who was there? What did they say? What were the circumstances around that interaction? For most of us, this goes back to family, and that's what makes this process so difficult. I don't blame my family for where I was before I started this journey; that's not the point here. The point is to be honest, raw, and vulnerable with yourself while you explore your past.

You can journal as we go, or you can simply close your eyes and think, but don't close your eyes while you're reading, okay? Think back to your relationships – friends, family, and romantic partners. In each relationship, how did you feel about yourself? I'm not asking how you feel (or felt) about the other person and there's a reason for that. This isn't about them; this is about you. How did you feel about yourself? Maybe you felt like shit most of the time because you chose relationships with people who were critical of you. Maybe you felt like you were constantly playing a game of "catch up" because you felt like nothing was ever enough. I'm sure you had some good relationships in there too, with people you felt comfortable enough with to let your guard down a little. Relationships with good people who made you laugh until your stomach hurt, and they didn't care that you snorted when you couldn't catch your breath from laughing so hard. I had those people too – only a few, but they were in there. I want you to remember the way you felt about yourself when you look back at these relationships because it says something about how you were treated and how comfortable (or uncomfortable) you were with each person.

One of my best friends, Jimmy, was the guitarist in the rock band I was in for over a dozen years. I've always loved music and had this dream of singing out with a rock band from a young age. This was super rebellious because I wasn't allowed to listen to rock music.

My sister and I used to sneak into the car and listen to the local rock station on the radio. I loved listening to bands like Led Zeppelin, Aerosmith, Journey, Mötley Crüe, Queen, and so many others. Other kids my age were going to New Kids On The Block concerts while I was content listening to rock music in the car.

After graduating from tech school with a music degree, I formed a few different bands. The one that lasted the longest was my favorite. I met Jimmy through another band member, Brad. Brad was also a good friend, and the bassist in our band. We had a ton of fun writing, playing, and just talking. I felt like I had known Jimmy my whole life after just a few months of hanging out. We would practice, drink, and shoot the breeze for hours. He was an amazing guy – a truly unique and special person.

For people looking from the outside in, he seemed rough around the edges. He was a biker, a hunter, and one of those guys you wouldn't mess with at the bar, but to me, he was a big teddy bear of a man. He was so kind to me and so genuine. We didn't agree on everything, but that didn't matter. He was one of the only people I've ever known who loved me unconditionally. We had a special brother/sister bond in a way I hadn't experienced with anyone else. Jimmy never judged me, even though he knew all my flaws and all my (many) imperfections. In 2014, Jimmy passed away in his sleep. I found out about his passing through social media, which isn't the way you want to find out that one of your best friends died. There isn't a good way to learn of a friend's passing, but social media makes it especially tough. No matter how close someone is to the deceased or how distant they are, everyone knows everything at the same time. There's no real time to digest the information before you receive messages from people asking what happened.

It was so surreal because I always thought he would be there. I thought he would meet my kids and be their cool uncle Jimmy. I thought we'd write music together forever and make weekend jam sessions a regular thing. Instead, he was just gone. Losing Jimmy was the hardest loss I had ever experienced, and I felt guilty for that. Losing my dad and my oldest sister should have been harder, right? I mean, what kind of daughter and sister feels worse about losing a friend than her family? Let me tell you something: you don't choose how you feel, and you do not need to apologize for your emotions.

After years of beating myself up for this, I came to realize that there was a reason why losing Jimmy hit me harder than my other losses: it was because of the way I felt in that relationship. I felt safe. I felt loved. I felt like I could say anything without having to worry about hurting his feelings. He knew where my heart was. I didn't have to overexplain everything or overanalyze anything because we had a "love me as I am, and I love you are you are" friendship. There were no conditions

– ever. He never tried to control what I did or what I said, and I was the same with him. I realize now that he was a one-of-a-kind gift in my life. He taught me that you can agree to disagree and still be cool with another person. He taught me that you should never have to prove your worth to anyone, and that anyone worth your while will make you feel that way. He taught me what true support looks like in a way I had never previously experienced.

This support is different from what you may receive from a lot of your friends. People like Jimmy are rare and special. You won't meet many of them, so when you do, it is important to recognize their value. These people need to be a part of your inner circle. How will you know if they support you? As you share your progress, you will see trends with people. Some may be excited for you, but a lot of people will back away. Why? Well, there are a number of reasons. For one, people are often threatened by success, feeling as if there is only a certain amount of success available and your success takes away from theirs. This couldn't be further from the truth. It's completely freaking ridiculous.

There are also people who will be straight-up jealous of you. That's a fact. People will throw shade your way and try to make you feel bad for your progress. Why are people so awful? You know, I don't have the answer to that question. Since I took control of my life, got in shape, set boundaries, and started saying no to whatever no longer serves my purpose, people have been particularly harsh. I've had people say some horrible things about me over the years, so I'm pretty familiar with harsh words. But you know what? It's okay. This shows their lack of character and has nothing to do with me.

CONSEQUENCES OF NOT SETTING BOUNDARIES

What happens if you don't set boundaries? What happens if you give in to all the guilt trips? What happens if you continue to allow toxic people to infiltrate your life? Well, as a result you will continue this cycle of being emotionally drained, unhealthy, and miserable. Those toxic people won't give a shit because it's easier to control you when you don't have self-esteem. You won't reach your goals and you won't even try to accomplish the things you want to do without boundaries. Will you lose weight and get fit? Nope, that won't happen. If it does, you will only keep the weight off until someone makes you feel bad for your success, at which point you'll self-sabotage, ending up back where you were before you started. The worst part is that you will teach your children that they can only be successful so long as they don't upset or outshine anyone. Without boundaries, your children will learn that as long as they stick within the social confines that have been handed down for generations, they will find success (as defined by those social confines), and they will learn this from your example.

I know that's not what you want. You are the one who is going to show your children that they can accomplish anything they want to achieve, so long as they are willing to do the work.

At this point, you know that you are in control of getting to where you want to be. You have the power to choose healthy relationships and set boundaries. People who criticize you, gossip about you, and undermine your success are not the people you want in your circle. It's better to have a few amazing, supportive, kind people close to you than it is to have a whole tribe of bullshit, backstabbing followers. When you know your value, you have no problem saying no to what no longer serves your purpose. I've given you the tools you need to block guilt trips, which breaks that negativity and creates the space you need to choose your own path.

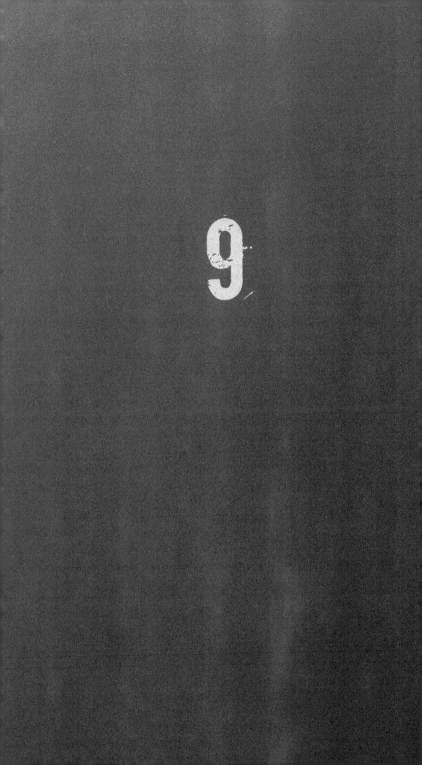

CHAPTER 9

"S" – SAYING HELL YEAH TO THE NEW YOU

CELEBRATE YOUR SUCCESS

Taking and sharing progress selfies has never been comfortable for me. It always feels a little off, but I share them anyway because celebrating your progress is one of the most important parts of your fitness journey. Laeti is one of my clients and close friends, and her fitness journey as a Badass Rebel Runner has been incredible. Not even a month into working out and adjusting her diet, she started feeling great. We grabbed coffee one day and I said, "Let me take a picture of you so you can see your progress."

She isn't great about taking progress selfies, so I knew I had to show her a side-by-side picture so she could see what I saw. I sent her the "before" and "after" pictures and she almost cried. She couldn't believe the difference. Her transformation was (and is) incredible. Seeing that progress picture motivated her to work even harder as she continues along her fitness journey. As her coach and as her friend, I am so proud of her. She is an inspiration for so many people, and she wears her title of being a Badass Rebel Runner with pride.

Since joining my program, her identity has completely changed. At the beginning of her fitness journey, Laeti was working a corporate job where she wasn't valued, and where her gifts and talents were not even acknowledged. Her confidence was so low that she didn't realize her worth. She felt stuck, as if that would forever be her life. I am so thrilled to share that she is no longer in that position. She gained confidence, acknowledged her self-worth, and built her business using her education and her passion for photography. She is living her best life, and is looking forward to her future as an entrepreneur. It all started with one decision; one choice. Like her, your best life awaits you. All it takes is one decision, one choice to take that first step forward.

You see, it is so important to celebrate your success and track your progress. You should be proud of yourself for all of the hard work you've put into your fitness journey – and don't ever let anyone tell you otherwise. Some people will celebrate your success, and others won't. I've had some pretty shitty responses to my progress shares, and that used to bother me. I felt like I had to respond and explain myself, validating my success. What the hell? No. When people respond negatively to your progress, it shows their lack of character and has nothing to do with you. It also shows that these people are not in a place of self-love. People who love themselves don't behave that way. For that matter, if you see a negative response from friends or family members, know that they don't support you. Supportive people don't behave that way. People who love you don't behave that way.

I started responding to criticism with this statement: "When you are ready to live your best life, I'm here to help." I wish them well and let them go. And you know what? These people stop – usually. The people who don't stand down are looking for a fight. They want an argument because they want to nitpick happy, successful people to take away that happiness and tear successful people down. Responding in alignment with my true self breaks that cycle of negativity.

I've also noticed how people respond to other people's progress/success stories. Some people are supportive, while others are not. Each day, I make an effort to like and/or comment on progress pictures and success stories. Whether they are my clients or not and whether I know them or not, I want to celebrate with anyone who has put the work into their health and well-being. You might think it's not important to do that, but it makes a difference in my opinion. Doing this spreads positivity to others, regardless of who they are, where they are, what they look like, or where they are in their journey. It is such a powerful, empowering action, and it takes a few minutes a day. You can choose to do this or not – that's completely up to you. I do encourage you to try it out because you will feel so awesome for being supportive of other people. Setting that example is a powerful tool in your own success.

TRACKING YOUR PROGRESS

When we think about weight loss, one of the most common ways of tracking success is the scale – that dreaded thing you've been tempted to throw out the window, that device you swear is never accurate, that number you don't want to see – the scale. You hate it, right? Most people who want to lose weight do despise it. You can definitely use your scale if you want to, but don't rely solely on your scale to track your progress or to measure your success. It is so easy to get super obsessed with the number you see, and that isn't healthy. If you want to weigh yourself as a way to track your progress, that's fine, but limit your weigh-ins to once a week. I'm serious; weigh yourself at the same time of day once each week and track that number. The rest of the week, I want you to forget about the scale. Your weight will fluctuate depending on the time of day, what you've had to eat and drink, your activity level, what you have going on in your life, your menstrual cycle, etc. So once each week, preferably at the beginning of the day before you have food, go ahead and weigh yourself, and that's it. Don't make me come take your scale away.

There are so many ways to track progress and I'd like you to step outside of your comfort zone. At the beginning of each week, take a full-body selfie – one from the front and one from the side. If you're talented enough to be able to take a selfie from the back, you go for it. I haven't gotten that one down yet. Hold on to these pictures and put them in an album labeled "progress pics" or "weekly selfies." It doesn't matter what you name the album, just label it so that you won't lose the pictures. What you'll notice is that week by week and month by month, your body will change. You will see real, noticeable changes as you compare these selfies side-by-side. This is one of the most motivating ways to track your progress because you can see your body changing. You will see your fat decrease, and you will see muscle definition take shape. You will see your legs and arms thin out, and even your face shape will change. When you look in the mirror each day, you won't notice these changes because you see yourself all the time. This is why it's so important to have these progress pictures, so you can look back and visually see your progress.

If you choose to share your progress pictures on social media (which I encourage you to do), take the first picture and put it side-by-side with your most current picture. This shows you, your friends, and your family how much progress you've made and how much work you've done to get there. Some people will support you, and those are the people you want in your circle. As for the people who don't support you? Wish them well and let them go. Maybe they'll be able to celebrate your success when they're in a place of self-love. It isn't your job to make them feel safe by minimizing your success. Stop that narrative right now. You celebrate the amazingness that is you and let them be.

For those of you who are number-centric and analytical, I know you need another way to track your success. You'll need a measuring tape for this one. At the beginning of each week, measure yourself and track these numbers (centimeters or inches – your choice). Measure your chest, waist, hips, thighs, and arms (around your bicep area). Week over week, you will see progress as these measurements decrease. During your major weight loss and fat burning phase, you will be surprised at how your actual size changes. It's incredible. Here's the thing – when you are done with the weight loss portion, some of you will want to focus on building muscle. As you build muscle, you may see a slight size increase in your chest, legs, and biceps, but that's normal. Don't freak out. What's amazing is that as you build muscle (which happens from the start of the process), you are helping your body burn fat. You will have strong muscle mass before you can see that definition, so please know that you are progressing more than you see and more than you can measure.

CELEBRATE YOUR SUCCESS

One part of this journey is a sense of accomplishment and pride. When you have a great workout, you are going to feel so amazing. Let that happen. Celebrate that feeling. When you see progress, you are going to get a little emotional, at least I did. In fact, I still do. I look at my side-by-side pictures and can't believe I ever looked like that "before" picture, but I'm so freaking proud of that woman. She was so unsure of herself and afraid of her success. The woman in the "before" pictures spent decades minimizing herself, her abilities, and her accomplishments to make other people comfortable. She was so lost, stuck, and hopeless, but she was brave. She said enough was enough and she decided to make a change. She stopped listening to other people and caring about feeding the egos of small-minded people. She found her "why," she made herself a priority, and she took that first step to start her fitness journey. I get emotional looking at her because I remember what it's like to feel that way, and I am so proud of that woman because she didn't take the easy way. She didn't settle. She started this journey and kept moving forward, one step at a time.

I used to try to shut off those feelings because I thought it was egotistical to be proud of myself. Please, don't even think that for a minute. You should be proud of yourself for each accomplishment you earn. Allow yourself to feel all the feels along the way. Be proud. Let that happen. If you get frustrated (which I know you will), let yourself feel those feels too. You've probably hidden your feelings for a long time. You've been upset, anxious, frustrated, sad, and angry – that's okay. Let yourself feel all of those emotions and use those feelings to cleanse your spirit. When you hide from your emotions, you disallow a whole part of you from existing. The more you block your emotions, the more those negative feelings take over. It's almost the opposite of what you'd think; you'd think that if you block your fear, anger, and sadness that you would only experience happiness and joy, but that's not how it works. When those negative emotions come to you, let them be. Don't let them stay too long- but give them space for a moment. Acknowledge them. Feel those feels, and then release them. Once you do that, you will start to feel more of that positive energy you crave.

SETTING YOU UP FOR SUCCESS BY SETTING EXPECTATIONS

During your fitness journey it is so important to allow yourself to heal and grow emotionally, just as much as you transform physically. You will be uncomfortable from time to time, and that's okay. That discomfort is a sign that you are growing and changing. People often want to stay in their comfort zone, and I get it. It feels safe there, but you aren't going to grow or become your most amazing self in your comfort zone, my friend. In a way, your physical transformation might be "easier" than the emotional and mental changes you experience. Yes, you will work your ass off physically, and it will be hard. Anyone who tells you differently is lying. You already know I don't bullshit you about anything; I give it to you straight. Why? Because I want you to be fully prepared for your journey. I want you to know what to expect, and it's just my personality, so know this – when we set expectations that are realistic, we are setting ourselves up for success.

WHAT DO YOU EAT, ANYWAY?

People always ask me what I eat. Well, I eat a lot. My decision to go vegan was about the animals. It was time for me to align my behavior with my beliefs – pretty simple. As I progressed in my fitness and health journey, I started moving toward a whole food, plant-based eating plan. What's interesting is that I thought I'd miss things like meat and cheese alternatives, but I don't, not even a little bit. Eliminating processed food has increased my performance and my energy level. Do I treat myself sometimes with vegan pizza or pie? You bet I do. I refuse to feel guilty for allowing myself a treat every now and again. I have zero guilt. Can you imagine feeling absolutely no guilt for eating something so decadent? Oh yeah, it's entirely possible. When you eat super healthy the vast majority of the time, it's okay to indulge sometimes. Not like eat-an-entire-large-pizza indulge, but more like, have a couple of pieces and you're good.

At the beginning of my week I meal prep, which usually involves quinoa, veggies, and either tofu or tempeh. I season the veggies and tofu/tempeh, pair it with the quinoa, and divvy it up for the week. That's lunch. For breakfast, I honestly love a banana and coffee because I'm not a huge breakfast eater. Dinner varies quite a bit because I like to mix it up. I make pasta, chili, soup, tacos, stir fry, spring rolls, whatever. I make sure it's vegan, organic, gluten-free, and as minimally processed as possible. There are so many delicious options that I've never felt unsatisfied with my food since eating vegan. Oh, did I mention snacks? I love potatoes – simple, delicious, versatile, and satisfying; they are so good. I also love making peanut butter protein balls with oats and dark chocolate. Yeah, just said that. Peanut butter and chocolate. Another favorite of mine are these amazing crispy buffalo cauliflower bites. They are so good and go over well at parties. Finish your day with some "nice" cream and you're all good. All of these recipes are a part of the Badass Rebel Runners program, in case you were wondering. Oh my word, I think I may have some cooking to do.

My point, now that you are hungry and want me to cook for you, is that you can love your food, do what is kind for the animals, do what is responsible for the environment, do what is healthiest for you, and always feel satisfied. How freaking amazing, right? Will people give you a rough time if you do choose to go vegan? Yeah, they probably will, but that has nothing to do with you, so wish them well and let them go. You don't have to justify your choices to anyone. Keeping these healthy meal and snack options on hand sets you up for success. Woo hoo! Delicious food? Check. Always feeling satisfied? Check. Giving your body the fuel it needs to thrive? Double check.

This journey will seem like work because it is. At the same time, you are going to learn to enjoy and embrace the work. You'll love the way you feel as you get fit and commit to eating healthy. You'll look at your progress pictures and smile because you're doing the work. You will have the energy you want – the energy you need – to play with your kids and be more active during your daily life. You'll want to do things that you were scared to try before. Enjoy this journey, every single bit of it. Allow yourself the space to enjoy this process. This is the journey that will change the course of your life. You are getting fit so you can show your children what a healthy woman looks like. Along the way, you are teaching them to have a healthy relationship with food and fitness. You are becoming the person you were always meant to be. Enjoy it. This is the good stuff, the fun part. This is the start of your new life – no turning back.

The importance of celebrating your success is something you will understand as you progress in your fitness journey. As you look back at your selfies (and measurements, weight, et cetera), you will feel such a sense of accomplishment. You know what? You are going to be so freaking proud of yourself, and I'm freaking proud of you, too. When you go all in and choose healthy food, good habits, and a positive mindset, you become unstoppable. You are going to enjoy trying delicious plant-based recipes, and I know you'll come up with some of your own. Learn to love food again. Learn to love yourself. Learn to celebrate your progress. I'm here to remind you of how amazing you are and how you deserve everything life has to offer. It's your time to shine.

10

"REBEL" – UNLEASH YOUR INNER BADASS REBEL

IT IS TIME TO UNLEASH OUR INNER BADASS REBEL

It's time, my dear. It is time for you to unleash your inner Badass Rebel. You have done the work to get to this point. You have a plan, and this time you aren't scared to take that step forward. You know it's all about progress and that perfection doesn't matter. You know that it is completely okay to make yourself a priority. In addition, now you know that you have to make time for yourself so that you can become the fit, healthy mom your children need. There is no turning back this time. You've had enough of feeling like you're not enough – you're done with that bullshit. You're done fearing change because you know that change leads to growth and growth is an important part of living a full life. You're ready. It's time.

This step is my favorite because you are so ready to be here, in this place. Close your eyes and take a deep breath. As you exhale, let go of your past self. Thank her for being brave enough to start this journey and tell her that you will think of her fondly as you look back on your progress. Tell her that you are okay, and she doesn't need to worry anymore. Tell her how amazing you feel and that you know you wouldn't be here without her. Thank her again. She has done what she needs to do and now you can let her go. She will always be a part of your story because she chose to take that first step. She knew you were waiting – she knew all along. She believed in you so much that she worked through her struggles, she conquered obstacles, and she kept moving forward, even when she had doubts. You will always be grateful to her and for her. It is time to move forward once more. One more deep breath in and let her be ever-present in the chapters of your story that have come to a close. Breathe out. Are you crying? I'm crying. That's okay, my dear because this is huge. Feel all those feels.

It is time for a new chapter.

You are writing your story right now and the most amazing part is that you are in control of what you write. This is your story and your life. You are in control of your destiny, and now that we've started this journey together, you are strong enough to accept nothing less than what you want from life. You aren't hiding anymore. You aren't settling. You no longer fear success. That last sentence is one of the most important lessons from this whole process, so let that sink in – you no longer fear success.

When you fear your own success, you shy away from doing anything that would pull you away from the crowd, but when you are no longer concerned with fitting in with the crowd, you shine. In a way, I was always worried about being successful because I knew people would shun me for it. I knew they would gossip, and I knew I would face backlash. I knew that if I succeeded – if I let myself shine – I wouldn't be accepted in some of the groups where I so desperately wanted to belong, and you know what? I was right. People do gossip about me. They throw shade. I get random messages about my success with questions about if I'm doing it right. People purposely try to discredit me and try to turn others against me. It sucks – kind of.

What I learned when people started pulling away from me is that there is so much freedom in distance. I felt lighter because these negative people, the ones who tried to make me feel guilty for my success and were actively trying to turn others against me, were no longer a part of my life. I let them go. They are not meant for me. Many of them tried to punish me by pushing away, but that was a gift. That space is exactly what I needed to become who I am today.

KNOW YOUR VALUE

Not too long ago, I had a moment of clarity. I was trying to prove my value to people without realizing I was doing it. I was doing all these things, making all the effort in relationships, and expecting that others would love and appreciate me. Instead, I felt so drained. I was exhausted from trying so hard to prove myself, so I stopped. You know, it could have been a painful moment, but it wasn't – I was liberated. I had more time and more space to do what I wanted to do. I had more time to invest in people who acknowledged my worth and appreciated my passion. Once again, that space has been a gift.

It is okay to let people go. You have been so conditioned to believe that you need to allow people to treat you however they choose, just because of their relation to you, how long you've known each other, how you met, et cetera. You already know what I'm going to say about that: it's all bullshit. If you feel like you have to prove your value to people, they don't love you. That's not what love looks like. If someone won't talk to you because they can't control you, they don't love you. That's not what love looks like. If someone gets pissed off because you are successful without their involvement, they don't love you. That's not what love looks like, either. Let that go. Those people aren't meant for you.

Darla, one of my newer clients, came to me with tears in her eyes and I already knew what she was going to say. She had posted a progress picture and a family member gave her a hard time for going vegan. This family member told Darla that she was "extreme" for choosing to eat plant-based and went on to say that she preferred Darla's "before" picture to her progress picture. Oh how I wanted to take that pain away from Darla because I know how deep that stings. I also wanted to contact that family member and give her a piece of my mind. But that isn't how you empower people.

Instead, I asked Darla to make a list of all the ways she feels better since starting her journey as a Badass Rebel Runner. Then I had her make a list of all the ways this family member contributed to these positive feelings. The first list was extensive. She felt confident for the first time in forever. She felt amazing in her clothes. She had more energy than she ever remembered having – even in her teens. This family member contributed absolutely nothing to these positive changes. Instead, they tried to undercut her success. I reminded Darla that this had nothing to do with her and everything to do with them. It showed their lack of character. She could respond, she could delete the comment, she could do nothing, or she could unfriend them.

A few weeks later I asked her what she chose to do about the situation. She defiantly told me (with a giggle) that she recommended the Badass Rebel Runners program to this family member who then promptly unfriended her. Darla found her voice, stood up for herself, and ended up eliminating one toxic relationship from her life. Since then, she has been a vocal supporter of other people who post progress pictures and encourages those who are working toward their goals. You see, when you know what it feels like to have "loved ones" treat you like shit, you want to show support and encouragement for others who are in that same position.

It is time for you to focus your energy on the people who matter – the people who love and support you. Instead of focusing on pleasing negative, toxic people, focus your energy on the positive people. These people understand that love is not about control, but rather about freedom. These people want you to succeed and want you to be happy. Your children are a part of your inner circle, obviously. Your spouse or partner, the friends and family you have who are supporting you, and the new friends and connections you will gain along this journey and beyond are the people who deserve your energy. All of these people are rallying behind you, so excited for you, happy to see your progress, and celebrating all of your success.

I can tell you right now that some of my favorite people are those who I've connected with only recently. They accept me for who I am and surprisingly have no issue with my edgy personality. That side of me was suppressed for so long because she didn't fit in with the crowd.

Screw fitting in with the crowd and every other limiting belief.

You were not born to fit in – you were born to shine.

If someone tries to dull your shine, you know that you need to let them go. Does this mean that you will say goodbye to these people forever? No, not necessarily. There may be people who need time to adjust to the new you. If they come back around with love and support, and without conditions, let them come back.

We need to surround ourselves with supportive people. Some may not come back around, and that's okay.

YOU DON'T OWE THEM ANYTHING

Something interesting happened along my journey – people tried to take credit for my success. I'm laughing right now because it's so ridiculous. Who does that? Who tries to take credit for something someone else does? As it turns out, a lot of people do this. In my case, there were a few select people who were guilty of this crappiness.

Here's how it happened – I did something cool and shared that success on social media. Let me backtrack for a minute; I told you about my list of things I want to accomplish before I turn forty, right? Okay, so I share my goals, progress, and success on social media in order to inspire others along my journey. This is all documented on my "See Jane Do Everything" account, and the goal is to show people that if a regular girl from Minneapolis, Minnesota, can crush all these goals and make extraordinary progress, they can do it too. I don't have special funding for this page. I don't have sponsors, and I don't have coaches, although I'll have to find specialty coaches for a couple of my goals. I'm not famous, and I don't have millions of followers. My hope is to inspire people by showing them that someone like me can achieve all of these goals by putting in the work. Anyway, after sharing some of these successes, I noticed a trend with certain people: they started talking about their role in my success.

Say what?

Yeah, these few people talked about how they used to support me way back when, years ago. They made comments about helping me with some random task, again, years ago. Listen, if I help you with something and you thank me, we're all good. You don't need to keep thanking me until the end of time. The same does not go for everyone, however, and these people had the idea, and the complex, that they had some sort of "right," or entitlement to my success. Keep in mind that they did not like anything I shared, nor had they been the least bit supportive in my journey. Still, they thought I owed them some fucked up debt of gratitude. Hell, no. I owed them nothing. When it comes to showing people gratitude for supporting me or helping me out, I'm good about thanking people – I mean good, too good. I show gratitude to the point of making people feel uncomfortable. You know that awkward hug you don't know if you should give? Yeah, I give that hug, every time. What about thanking people profusely for help and support? Yep, that's also me. Guess who is sending a case of beer or a hotdish to someone for doing something nice? Yes. It's the right thing to do. I know damn well that if someone helped me or supported me in any way, I thanked them, showed gratitude, and either gave them food or an awkward hug, and that's enough. Once you thank someone, you're good. You don't owe them anything else.

You will probably have an experience similar to mine, although I hope you don't. If you do, please don't feel like you need to call this person up and thank them, yet again, for something they did years ago. Do you know what is happening on a deeper level? These people can't handle that you succeeded without their involvement. The thing is, you are successful because they are not involved in the process. Toxic people will try to drag you down, make you feel guilty, and try to take credit for your success. Wish them well and let them go. You're done with that shit.

GIVE YOUR ENERGY WISELY

You are vibrating on a different level now. That energy is who you are. You'll notice that people who have the same energy as you (people vibrating on the same level), will make you feel great about yourself, your success, and what lies ahead. On the flip side, you will notice that people on a lower vibration will drain your energy. They'll say things to dismiss your success or to question why you're doing what you're doing. Do you remember what I told you to do in these situations? Put up your hand and say, "Fuck that." People who are on a lower vibration than you will try to drain your energy and pull you down to their level. They think that if you are successful, they can't be, as if there's a limited amount of success in the world and you're taking their share. Um, no, that's not how it works. You already know this. When you notice people acting this way, you may need to limit your time with these people. In some cases, they may not be for you anymore; you have the ability to navigate that as you go. The main takeaway is that if you spend time with people, they need to match your energy.

SUPPORT LIKE YOU WANT TO BE SUPPORTED

We talked about surrounding yourself with people who support you, and now we need to chat about how you will be that person for others. It's simple: pay it forward and be supportive. Be the person you so badly needed during your journey. Give someone a "like" on social media, congratulate their progress, or offer positive words of encouragement. When you see someone struggling, let them know they are progressing through that struggle. Lift people up. Encourage them and support them. You will be amazed at how great you feel. When you share positive energy with others, it regenerates ten times over within you. You lose nothing and gain so much. Those people will remember you and your support and encouragement. In my experience, they will share that same positive energy with others. There is no limit to the amount of good, positive energy you can put out into the world, so do it. Be that uplifting person. Be that person who reacts with kindness and compassion. Don't let the negative crap you see out there drag you down or make you feel like your acts of kindness won't matter. They do. That positivity is contagious, and people will be so grateful for your support. I know negativity is more popular. Positivity leads to better results. Trust me.

CREATE SHORT-TERM AND LONG-TERM GOALS

Part of this process is to set your short-term and long-term goals. Maybe you want to run a 5k or even a marathon. Perhaps your goal is to follow your passion and create something amazing. Whatever it is you want to do, have a plan. As you work through your plan, celebrate the little wins. Remember that each step forward is exactly that; you don't achieve goals in one giant leap. Success takes work, persistence, and patience. For your short-term goals, you want to consider the next one to six months. What do you want to accomplish? From a fitness standpoint, you are ready to create a goal for yourself. That 5k is a great one.

For your long-term goals, you want to look at anything beyond that six-month mark. Sometimes it helps to have a long-term goal that is a little further out. My example of both types of goals is the list that I gave myself two years to accomplish. Some of the items were short-term goals and some were long-term goals, but having that list motivated me to keep moving forward with my fitness, my creativity, and my passion. Think about it and don't be afraid of what comes to mind. Embrace these ideas because there's a reason why you want to do these things. That's your Badass Rebel challenging you to live your best life.

CREATE SPACE TO SIMPLY BE

We've talked a lot about doing quite a number of things, and as much as I love to crush goals, it is equally important to create the time and space to exist in your own space. Unplug from social media for the weekend;

put your phone down and play with your children. Instead of screen time, have reading time. Be fully present in each moment, with no secondary noise in the background. Maybe you like to meditate. If you do, commit to it. Stop looking at your phone every two seconds. I read a study that said spending as little as ten minutes outside, with no electronic devices, improves your mental health. I believe it because it's easy to get caught up in doing so much that we forget to make time to simply be. Create that space and be fully present. Make time to not be so busy. When you let yourself be, you recharge your battery so that when you get back to crushing your goals, you have more energy to make it happen. It's pretty awesome, trust me.

Your Badass Rebel self is here to stay. You know that there is no "plan B." This is you, doing what you've always wanted to do. You've been capable this whole time. Sure, you needed a little push, and yeah, you needed someone to show you how it's done, but you already had the strength to get here. It took you a little while to discover that about yourself, but it's been there for a long time. Now you have the power to keep moving forward. You know that you will face obstacles because that's how life works, but you also know that you will conquer every obstacle you face. Your inner

Badass Rebel is here to stay, and you are a shining example of what a fit, healthy mom looks like. Never again will you shy away from success or dim your shine. You were not born to live an ordinary life. You were born to be extraordinary – an extraordinary Badass Rebel.

This new version of you knows your value. You understand that in order to create the life you want, you need to let go of who you used to be. Your energy is so focused on what you are going to accomplish that you no longer waste time on anything that does not serve your purpose. Setting short-term and long-term goals will help you continue to move forward with a clear vision of the path meant for you. As obstacles arise, you know you will smash the shit out of them because that's what Badass Rebel Runners do. Now that you're in this place, you know that this time is different. There is no stopping. Quitting is no longer an option. You will continue to move forward, each and every day.

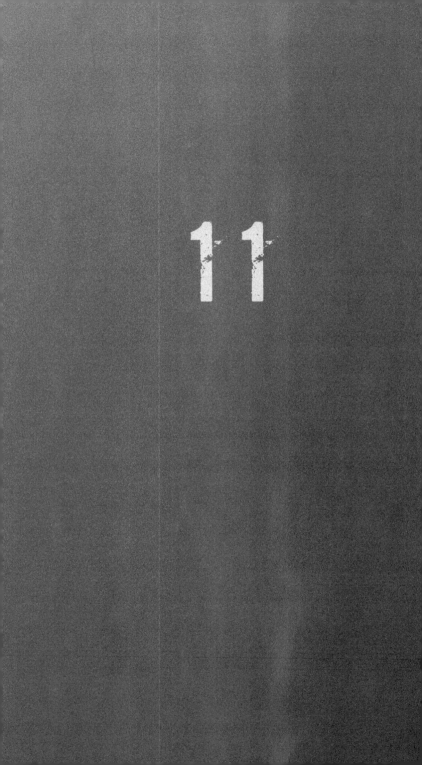

CHAPTER 11

BUT...WHAT IF?

Y ou have everything you need to work your way through this process, but you still have questions. I get it. Of course, you have questions. This is the last weight loss/fitness/health program you're ever going to need, as long as you stick with it and do the work. Yeah, okay Jane, you're thinking, but what if I don't have what it takes to do this? You absolutely have what it takes to this, to follow through, and to unleash your inner Badass Rebel. You wouldn't have chosen this book if you didn't have what it takes. You made the decision to change your life the moment you ordered the book. You decided you were ready the second you started reading it. The fact that you made it all the way through to the end shows me how bad you want it and how much you want to change. I know that you are so freaking ready this time, unlike all those other times. This time you know your purpose; you know what to do because I've given you everything you need. It's all right here.

WHAT HAPPENS IF I SCREW UP?

Everyone screws up. That's a part of life. I guarantee you that you have a 100 percent probability of screwing up at multiple points along your journey. Here's the secret about those moments that no one seems to understand – those are some of the most beautiful, meaningful parts of your journey. Why? Because, my dear, when you screw up and show that you are indeed human, you have the ability to show your resolve. You have this wonderful opportunity to rise up, learn from your screw up, and keep moving forward. Embrace these moments as they come instead of hiding from them. That's the difference between people who succeed and people who are too afraid to succeed.

BUT WHAT IF I DON'T HAVE TIME?

Don't even come at me saying, "I don't have time." Yes, you do – you absolutely have time to make yourself a priority. You have time to show your children what it looks like to value yourself, and you have time to make healthy choices each day. We all have the same amount of time in a day, but what you do with that time is up to you. Allocating your time in a way that best serves you may require you to change things up a little bit. Let's say you have a job outside the home. What do you do on your lunch break? Is it serving your purpose?

Here's what I mean: I used to go on my lunch break and chat with my coworkers. Without fail, the conversation would lead to complaints about work, spouses, obligations, money, et cetera. I would go back to my desk more exhausted than before my break. I realized that the healthiest thing for me to do on my lunch break was to detach from work altogether. I'd take my phone and headphones and go for a walk while listening to music, instead of talking with my coworkers. They weren't super happy that I stopped being a "team player" at lunch, but there wasn't any real team building happening in those interactions anyway. I chose to do something that helped me unwind, refresh, and reenergize during that time. Your situation might be different. Maybe you're starting your own business (or you're already a business owner) and your lunch time is when you connect with people and network for your business. That is a fantastic use of your time, so don't stop doing that; it is serving your purpose well. My point is, you have time, but it's all about how you use it.

WHAT IF I GET PUSHBACK FROM MY FAMILY AND FRIENDS?

I want to tell you honestly that you will get pushback. People will try to make you feel guilty for making time to take care of yourself, but you already know what to do when this happens. Hold up your hand and say, "Fuck that." Say, "Screw that," or whatever it is you choose to say to break that negative energy. People will absolutely give you a hard time. Some won't understand what you're doing and won't support you. As much as it sucks, it shows you something super important. You learn who has your back. I've been at this for quite a while and I still get pushback from family and friends. They question why I eat a whole food, vegan diet or why I run so much. People give me crap for being fit. These same people said nothing about my looks, weight, or health when I was obese. They never showed concern for my health when there was something to be concerned about. This is how some people work; they feel comfortable with things the way they are and aren't comfortable with change.

There are also people who will be jealous of your progress and your success. They would rather see you overweight and unhealthy because it makes them feel better about their situation. Others want you to stay uncomfortable and miserable because they feel like they shine brighter when your flame is dim. They like that you feel so awful because it makes them feel superior. As you progress through this journey, pay attention to all of these things because you will learn a lot about the people around you. When people have a negative reaction to your progress and your success, it shows their lack of character and has nothing to do with you. You are done minimizing yourself to feed the egos of the weak.

WHAT IF I DO ALL THIS WORK AND DON'T SEE RESULTS?

That isn't possible. When you do the work, you will see results. The Badass Rebel Program is here for you to set you up for success. The reason why I shared different ways of measuring and tracking your progress is to help you see your results, regardless of which tracking type works for you. You already know your weight loss won't happen overnight. We're done with the quick fix bullshit; quick fixes never work, and you've wasted enough time and money on that crap. This time is different because it is not a quick fix, a fad diet, or an over-promise-under-deliver program. No, this is a lifestyle. You will see results and you will maintain these results. This time, you have fully committed to doing the work so you can teach your children how to have a healthy relationship with food and fitness. There is no going back. You know what's behind you, and there is no way in hell you're going to return to that place. From this point forward, you are going to progress, overcome, and succeed.

WHY IT IS SO IMPORTANT TO FULLY COMMIT TO THIS PROGRAM, YOURSELF, AND YOUR FUTURE

Think of where you want to be six months from now. Now envision yourself one year from now, two years, or five years in the future. You want to be in shape and be healthy so you can show your children what a healthy woman looks like. Moreover, you want to teach your children how to have a healthy relationship with food and fitness. You want to break the cycle you've seen repeated so many times in your life and in your family. Committing to the Badass Rebel Program means you are actively choosing to say, "yes" to the fit, healthy role model you want to be for your children. The future you've envisioned depends on what you choose to do today. You can do nothing and stay exactly where you are, but I know that's not what you want. You're done with feeling helpless about your situation. I know where you have been, and you are sick and tired of being so freaking tired. You've had enough of feeling like you're not enough. You are ready to do the work and become who you are meant to be.

When I started this journey, I had no idea how I was going to get to where I wanted to be, but I knew the direction I needed to go. It was all new territory. I had never committed to my health before. I never understood my value. I felt as though self-care was selfish, at least for me. I felt as though I didn't deserve to live the life I wanted to live. Once I fully committed to this journey, things changed. I did the work, day in and day out. I still do. When you're fit, that isn't the end of your journey. This is a complete lifestyle change, not a one and done. My attitude changed. I started believing in myself and I stopped hiding my personality that had always been "too much" for some people. I embraced my Badass Rebel, my edge, and my feistiness. As my journey progressed, opportunities presented themselves, and this time, I wasn't afraid to say yes. If you want to accomplish something you've never achieved, you need to do what you've never done. With that in mind, I stopped allowing fear to block my progress. Instead of hiding from fear, I acknowledged it for exactly what it was in each situation. I allowed it to have that space for a moment, and then I let it go. Doing this has afforded me opportunities I could have only dreamed of before.

Why have these opportunities presented themselves this time around? I made the commitment to do what I had never done in order to accomplish the things I had yet to achieve. This completely changed my mindset, and the same will happen for you. You will see opportunities where you never thought to look before. Your future self – that fit, healthy mom – is waiting for you to take that first step, so when you look back on this moment six months or one year from now, you will thank yourself for being brave enough to make this first and most important step.

12

ONE MORE THING BEFORE YOU GO

G one are the days when you allowed yourself to feel like complete and utter shit. Gone are the days when you allowed yourself to feel hopeless about your situation, and gone are the days when you had no idea how to get fit and healthy. You know that you are not stuck where you are. You know that you have the power to change your life. The Badass Rebel Program is here to show you how to get fit and to motivate you along the way. Your journey is going to be amazing and I am so proud of you for believing in yourself enough to get started.

I've given you all the tools you need to achieve success. For starters, you know how to find your "why." My guess is that you already knew this part, but you just needed a reminder. You've done the work to uncover the reasons why you've failed in the past, which means you won't go down that road again. You know your responsibility in this process. It's all you, my friend. No one else's opinion of your journey matters. You know what you want, and this time, you're not letting anyone deter you from your goals. I've given you a roadmap of what to do in order to achieve sustainable results. This isn't like all those other times because this time you're committing to a healthy lifestyle.

The toxic relationships that held you back in the past have run their course. Now you have the power to wish them well and let them go. This process is about so much more than weight loss. This process goes deep to empower you to create real, lasting, sustainable changes as you become the most authentic version of yourself.

Now it's time for my favorite part; it's time for me to share what I see for you once you complete the Badass Rebel Program.

You will be empowered, fearless, strong, brave, and fierce.

For the first time, you will embrace your authenticity. You will embrace your inner Badass. You will have the courage to let go of toxic people, relationships, and situations so you can shine the way you were meant to, without hesitation. You will embrace your strength, become your authentic self, and find your awesome. You will let go of fear – the fear of failure, the fear of other people's expectations, the fear of isolation, and the fear of screwing it all up. You will be healthy in mind, body, and spirit. You will finally release the stress and worry that you've carried for so long. I know how much that's weighed you down, and you've held onto it for far too long, my friend. You will be fearless as you set your goals and courageous in your pursuit of success.

For those of you who have experienced personal loss, I want you to know that it's okay to be sad and miss the ones you've lost. It's also okay to keep moving forward and live your best life because this is how you honor those who have passed on.

You have what you need to complete this journey, and you can do this all on your own. I've given you everything you need to succeed. This time is different because you're ready. This time is different because you have a blueprint to follow from someone who has been there, done the work, and succeeded. This time is different because you know it's not just about the weight. This time is different because you are different.

You are amazing. You are strong. You are fierce. You are capable of accomplishing anything you want to achieve, as long as you are willing to do the work. You are done playing small to make others feel big. You are done minimizing your value because now you know your worth. It is time to unleash your inner Badass Rebel because she has been waiting for you to be ready. Now that you're here in this place, ready to embrace your most authentic self, you know that you will never dim your light again. Shine on, do the work, and keep moving forward. You've got this.

Remember – you were not born to live an ordinary life. You were born to be extraordinary.

ACKNOWLEDGMENTS

My daughter Reagan, my love, my light, my favorite human being, and my "why" for everything I do. You inspire me to be a better mom and a stronger woman with each passing day. May you always be fearless in the pursuit of your dreams. The world need you to be completely, unapologetically who you are- no holding back. You were born to shine, my love.

My husband, my best friend, steadfast partner, and the best father I could have chosen for our daughter. Thank you for giving me freedom to pursue my dreams. Your support, love, and understanding inspire me to keep moving forward. As we journey on together, I know that while our story has been incredible, our best years are yet to come.

My mom, my closest friend and most trusted advisor. Thank you for loving me unconditionally, supporting me even when I didn't know which direction I was heading, and encouraging me to pursue my true calling. You believed in me even when I didn't believe in myself, and I am forever grateful. You are braver than you know, and you inspire me to be fearless.

My four-legged cheering squad (Zoe, Roscoe, and in loving memory of Noah), my sweetest, most understanding, furriest kiddos. Thank you for reminding me to stop and enjoy the little things. Your zest for life keeps me grounded and lifts my spirit each day. Your silliness and quirkiness reminds me of the beauty that comes from being unique. Thank you for warming my feet and my heart. Your unconditional love, nose nudges, and kisses are a few of my favorite things.

The Incubated Author Team: Cory, my editing angel and my spirit animal, you are extraordinary. Thank you for helping me speak my truth through my book and having fun while doing the work. Cheyenne, my guide throughout this process, and question-answering queen. Thank you for having all the answers. Mehrina, my starting line, thank you for helping me focus my energy exactly where it needed to be in order to start this project.

Dr. Angela Lauria, the life force and fierce guardian of all that is unique, creative, and beautiful. Thank you for creating this space for all of us misfits. What was once broken, battered, and bruised is now put back together to create the most beautiful vision of strength.

This space is held by those who are brave enough to embrace their flaws, create imperfect perfection, and those who understand that true power comes from never fitting in with the crowd. You inspire me to be exactly who I'm meant to be and to make the difference I was born to make.

To the Vegan community who are good friends and some of my most amazing supporters: thank you for being fearless as you stand up for those who cannot speak for themselves. Thank you for inspiring people to challenge the status quo. Your strength, compassion, and kindness are changing the world, one person at a time, one interaction at a time. You are a light in a world full of darkness and I am forever grateful for each and every one of you. Keep shining.

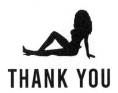

THANK YOU

Thank you so much for making the time to read my book. Now that you are here, you are already on your way to creating the life you deserve. As a mentor and coach, I want to do what I can to help you along your journey.

For exclusive access to my popular Badass Rebel class, simply email me to receive the link. Email badassrebelrunners@gmail.com with the subject line: ***Badass Rebel Master Class.***

I am passionate about helping people just like you and look forward to sharing in your journey. I am sending you so much love, strength, and all the badassery you need to continue to move forward.

Stay fierce,

Jane Elizabeth (Coach Jane)

www.badassrebelrunners.net

www.facebook.com/badassrebelrunners

www.facebook.com/seejanedoeverything

www.instagram.com/badass.rebel.runners

www.instagram.com/see.jane.do.everything

ABOUT THE AUTHOR

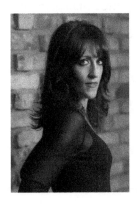

JANE ELIZABETH is a certified personal trainer and life coach who teaches women how to get in shape, stay in shape, and live a healthy, sustainable lifestyle. After suffering a series of losses and hardships, Jane found herself overweight, unhealthy, and unhappy. Once her daughter was born, Jane realized that she needed to be the example she wanted her daughter to emulate.

Jane began a journey into health and fitness, where she fought her way to a healthy lifestyle, losing eighty pounds and becoming a strong, fit, powerful, badass mom.

After spending the better part of two decades working in sales, management, and human resources, Jane left her corporate job and became a certified personal trainer and life coach, and created the Badass Rebel Runners Program. Through her unique blend of one-on-one coaching, her mobile app, and motivational speeches, Jane motivates, inspires, and supports her clients as they work through her program and become fit, healthy, and empowered.

In her corporate years, Jane earned an undergraduate and graduate degree in human resource management. After changing her focus to serving others, Jane earned certifications as a personal trainer and life coach.

Originally from Minnesota, Jane is a California girl at heart. She loves the outdoors, the beach, sunshine, music, and long-distance running. She resides with her husband, daughter, and three senior rescue dogs in a house that always feels like home to whomever drops by for a home-cooked meal.

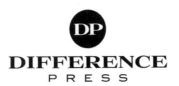

ABOUT DIFFERENCE PRESS

Difference Press is the exclusive publishing arm of The Author Incubator, an educational company for entrepreneurs – including life coaches, healers, consultants, and community leaders – looking for a comprehensive solution to get their books written, published, and promoted. Its founder, Dr. Angela Lauria, has been bringing to life the literary ventures of hundreds of authors-in-transformation since 1994.

A boutique-style self-publishing service for clients of The Author Incubator, Difference Press boasts a fair and easy-to-understand profit structure, low-priced author copies, and author-friendly contract terms. Most importantly, all of our #incubatedauthors maintain ownership of their copyright at all times.

LET'S START A MOVEMENT WITH YOUR MESSAGE

In a market where hundreds of thousands of books are published every year and are never heard from again,

The Author Incubator is different. Not only do all Difference Press books reach Amazon bestseller status, but all of our authors are actively changing lives and making a difference.

Since launching in 2013, we've served over 500 authors who came to us with an idea for a book and were able to write it and get it self-published in less than 6 months. In addition, more than 100 of those books were picked up by traditional publishers and are now available in book stores. We do this by selecting the highest quality and highest potential applicants for our future programs.

Our program doesn't only teach you how to write a book – our team of coaches, developmental editors, copy editors, art directors, and marketing experts incubate you from having a book idea to being a published, bestselling author, ensuring that the book you create can actually make a difference in the world. Then we give you the training you need to use your book to make the difference in the world, or to create a business out of serving your readers.

ARE YOU READY TO MAKE A DIFFERENCE?

You've seen other people make a difference with a book. Now it's your turn. If you are ready to stop watching and start taking massive action, go to http://theau-thorincubator.com/apply/.

"Yes, I'm ready!"

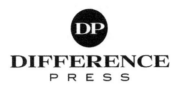

DIFFERENCE
P R E S S

OTHER BOOKS
BY DIFFERENCE PRESS

So You Just Found out You're a Healer: Uncover Your Psychic and Healing Gifts by Marlo Andersen

Millionaire Business Culture: 7 Steps to Create an All-Star Team to Help You Grow Your Business, Work Less, and Enjoy What You Do More by Lina Betancur

Fulfilled: Thrive as a Female Physician by Helen Blake, MD

Be Strong, Be Wise in the Age of #MeToo: The College Student's Guide to Sexual Safety by Amy R. Carpenter

The Spirit Connection: The Bereaved Parent's Guide to Moving beyond the Grief and Communing with Your Child by Erin E. Chandler

To Pee or Not to Pee?: The Guide to Reducing and Eliminating Urinary Incontinence by Shelia Craig Whiteman PT, DPT, CLT

Help! My Loved One Has Cancer: 8 Steps to Prevent Caregiver Burnout by Josephine Grace

Pelvic Pain Game Changer: 6 Steps to a Healthier You by Carolyn Marthanóir

Intimate Partnership: The Essential Guide to Feeling Sexy, Connected, and Whole by Katherine McClelland

Why Do Contractors Lie?: The Investor's Guide to Hire for Success by J.O.A. Maurice

Burnout Bible: The Nursing Career Survival Guide by Brooke Shepard DNP, HWNC-BC

Piecing Your Heart Back Together: The Roadmap to Healing and Thriving after a Breakup or Divorce by Carmen Silvestro

How to Get over Being Humiliated: Starting over after Losing Your Career by Leesa Ward

Healing the Wounds of Divorce: How to Move on Healthier, Happier, and More Fulfilled by Freda R. Wilson